## THE NATURAL WAY SERIES

Increasing numbers of people worldwide are falling victim to illnesses which modern medicine, for all its technical advances, seems often powerless to prevent – and sometimes actually causes. To help with these so-called 'diseases of civilization' more and more people are turning to 'natural' medicine for an answer. The *Natural Way* series aims to offer clear, practical and reliable guidance to the safest, gentlest and most effective treatments available – and so to give sufferers and their families the information they need to make their own choices about the most suitable treatments.

*Other titles in the* Natural Way *series*

Allergies
Arthritis & Rheumatism
Asthma
Back Pain
Chronic Fatigue Syndrome
Colds & Flu
Cystitis
Diabetes
Eczema
Heart Disease
HIV & Aids
Infertility
Irritable Bowel Syndrome
Migraine
Multiple Sclerosis
Premenstrual Syndrome
Psoriasis

THE NATURAL WAY

# Cancer

*Philip Barron*

*Series medical consultants*
*Dr Peter Albright MD (USA)*
*& Dr David Peters MD (UK)*

Approved by the
AMERICAN HOLISTIC MEDICAL ASSOCIATION
& BRITISH HOLISTIC MEDICAL ASSOCIATION

E L E M E N T
Shaftesbury, Dorset ● Rockport, Massachusetts
Melbourne, Victoria

© Element Books Limited 1996
Text © Philip Barron 1996

First published in the UK in 1996 by
Element Books Limited
Shaftesbury, Dorset SP7 8BP

Published in the USA in 1996 by
Element Books, Inc.
PO Box 830, Rockport, MA 01966

Published in Australia in 1996 by
Element Books
and distributed by
Penguin Books Australia Limited
487 Maroondah Highway, Ringwood, Victoria 3134

Reissued 1998

Cover design by Slatter-Anderson
Designed and typeset by Linda Reed and Joss Nizan
Printed and bound in in Great Britain

British Library Cataloguing in Publication
data available

Library of Congress Cataloging in Publication Data
Young, Pat.
Cancer/Pat Young.
p.   cm. -- (Natural way )
Includes bibliographical references and index.
ISBN 1–85230–799-4 (pb: alk. paper)
1. Cancer–Alternative treatment. 2. Holistic medicine.
3. Naturopathy. I. Title. II. Series: Natural way series.
RC271.A62Y68 1996
616.99'4–dc20        96–12362
CIP

ISBN 1 85230 799 4

# Contents

# Illustrations

To the memory of CWS 'Cubby' Thomas
for whom this book came too late to be of any help
but in the hope that it may help others

## Acknowledgements

Thanks for help in various ways are gratefully extended to Dr Rosy Daniel, medical director of the Bristol Cancer Help Centre, UK, the series' medical consultants Dr Peter Albright and Dr David Peters, healer and counsellor Barbara Siddall, independent researcher Hans R Larsen, the *International Journal of Alternative & Complementary Medicine*, and its editor Graeme Millar, and especially to series editor Richard Thomas without whom this book would not have happened.

# Introduction

Cancer is probably the most feared of all diseases, even though nearly twice as many people in the Western world die of heart disease than 'the Big C'. This reputation is as much due to the mysterious and still largely unknown cause of most of the many forms of cancer as to modern medicine's inability so far to find a cure for the most serious and common cancers. The disease appears to strike at random and be a virtual death sentence for anyone unfortunate enough to become afflicted.

But this is not quite the true story.

Not only has conventional medicine itself moved on in its understanding and treatment of the disease – so that some types of cancers can now be treated and cured completely if caught early enough – but people's frustration with medicine's apparent lack of success with the commoner types has resulted in a wide range of alternative treatments being developed and tried.

Some of these treatments have turned out to be worthless but others, particularly those concentrating on healthy eating and living, have produced so much success that pioneering cancer specialists in almost all Western countries are now taking a long and serious look at how much and how far to include them in the routine treatment of cancer patients.

Conventional medicine and the so-called 'natural therapies' are likely to see a greater interdependence and coming together in the future and nowhere is this more likely than in the treatment and care of cancer. The result is that it is now virtually certain that the treatment of cancer in the future will not be that of the past. And that is good news for anyone suffering from this most disturbing and insidious of diseases.

People worldwide are looking harder than ever for treatments that are as gentle as they are safe and effective. *The Natural Way: Cancer*, as well as covering the conventional approaches to cancer, introduces you to those 'gentle treatments', many of them coming under the heading of natural medicine.

Natural therapies cannot – or should not – claim to cure cancer, any more than can conventional medicine. But many of those included in this book have been shown to play a significant, even central, part for some people in helping to alleviate and sometimes reduce many of the symptoms of the disease, particularly when used in combination. Above all, studies show they can improve the quality and length of life.

Therapies such as massage, nutrition, relaxation, aromatherapy, meditation, visualization and counselling are just some of the examples of the approaches that anyone with cancer can safely turn to. They can be confident that their chances of seeing an improvement are high if they take the decision to help themselves, act soon enough and make sure the therapists they see are qualified, experienced and responsible people.

Cancer is a hard one to beat but it *is* possible – without drugs or surgery and without expecting a miracle. This book tells you what to look for in the quest for the safest, gentlest and most effective treatment for cancer, where to look for it and how to get it.

# CHAPTER 1

# What is cancer?

*How it develops, who and what it affects and what to look for*

Cancer is a disease in which the cells of the body go out of control and start growing unchecked and independently of the rest of the body. Like so many vandals on the rampage, they rebel against the body's normal 'rules' and form their own breakaway organizations.

These rebel organizations or 'growths' then start interfering with the way the body works and, if nothing is done to stop them, cause the failure of important organs and lead to death.

The reasons why cells go berserk like this are many and complicated and not yet fully understood. It seems to be a combination of both internal factors such as diet and individual psychology, and external conditions such as environmental pollution. It's this largely unknown nature of cancer that makes it feared by so many – coupled with the fact that treatment is often difficult and dangerous and cure still uncertain and unpredictable in most cases.

The main theories about how and why cells first turn against the body are explained in chapters 2 and 3. But we do at least know what happens once cancer has started.

## How cancer develops

Cancer develops in three stages:

● First, diseased cells grow and establish themselves in a particular part of the body, infiltrating the tissues around them. Cancer in this original site is known as a 'primary cancer'. (More details about the very early stages of the develoment of cancer can be found in chapter 2.)

● Next, they move to a nearby gland (called a *lymph node*), which is part of the body's immune or defence system, and from there they travel to other parts of the body.

● Diseased cells lodge themselves in these 'secondary' sites and start to grow again, often very quickly, invading the area around them aggressively. Cancers in these secondary sites are known as 'secondary cancers'. (It is this apparently sideways or 'crab-like' movement of the cancerous cells that gives cancer its name. Cancer comes from the Latin word for 'crab'.)

## The different terms used in cancer

The full complexity of the disease we call 'cancer' is only really understood when we realize that cancer is not one disease but over 200. This is because there are more than 200 different cells in the human body and cancer affects each one differently.

To sort out the different types doctors have invented their own language to describe them. To begin with, an abnormal growth of any kind may be called a 'tumour' or a *neoplasm* ('neo' simply means 'new', and 'plasm' means 'form'). So an illness arising is a *neoplastic disorder*.

If the tumour or growth is harmless it will be described as 'benign'. A benign growth does not spread to the tissue around it so that it does no damage. It just sits there doing no particular good but no harm either. Examples of benign growths are warts, cysts and polyps.

A 'malignant' growth is a different matter altogether. It cannot be contained and continues to spread unchecked so that it damages the area where it started before moving on to damage new areas in other parts of the body. Cancer is a malignant growth.

Different medical terms are given to cancers growing in different parts of the body:

- *Carcinoma* is cancer of what is known as *epithelial* tissue – the skin covering the outside of the body and the mucous membrane lining the cavities inside. This is by far the most common type of cancer and includes cancers of the breast, lung, colon, prostate and skin.
- *Sarcoma* is cancer of the bones, tendons and muscles.
- *Lymphoma* is cancer of the glands (or 'nodes') or other sections of the *lymphatic system*. The lymphatic system is part of the body's defence or 'immune system' (see chapter 2).
- *Leukaemia* is cancer of the blood.

Cancers that spread to other sites are described by the medical term *metastasis* – and so cancers that move from the original area to a second area are said by doctors to *metastasize to* that area. So, for example, a primary cancer in the breast may produce a secondary growth or metastasis in the bones or lungs, cancer of the lungs may metastasize to the brain and bone marrow, and cancer of the liver may be a metastasis of a cancer that started in the colon.


## Early warning signs of cancer

Early detection of all types of cancer is vitally important. People should be continually vigilant for unusual changes in the body that might mean a cancer is starting to grow. The following are the common early warning signs of cancer:

- a lump or thickened tissue in the breast, testicles, or any other part of the body
- a sore or ulcer that will not heal
- persistent hoarseness or a nagging cough with blood
- persistent abdominal pain, large lumps in the abdomen or difficulty in swallowing
- changes in your bowel or bladder habits
- obvious changes in a wart or mole
- unusual bleeding or discharge
- unexpected weight loss or loss of appetite
- undue fatigue, lassitude, or malaise
- persistent pain (though cancer is not always painful)
- painless, swollen glands that remain enlarged

None of these signs means cancer is definitely there. They could all be symptoms of a 'benign' condition that can be quickly and easily cleared up with the right treatment. But in case one of them is an early warning of cancer you should go and tell your doctor straight away. No responsible health professional should fail to take you seriously, examine you carefully, and refer you to a specialist if he or she thinks there is anything that needs to be investigated further.

*Don't worry about bothering your doctor unnecessarily. A good doctor should be pleased that you are being careful about your health and even more pleased to be able to tell you that your condition can be successfully treated. Equally, if your doctor does suspect something sinister is going on he or she should be just as glad to refer you for further investigations as soon as possible so that you have the best possible chance of cure by the gentlest, safest and most effective methods available.*

## The different sorts of cancer

Cancer differs from country to country and from region to region. Not every country registers the types of cancer cases occurring each year so it is difficult to give accurate statistics. But it is clear that some types of cancer are commoner in Western countries like America and Britain than in Eastern countries such as Japan or so-called 'developing' countries like Africa.

In Japan, for example, there are many more cases of stomach cancer than there are in the West, and in Africa liver cancer is much more widespread than elsewhere.

Overall, though, the ten most common cancers found worldwide seem to be of the lung, stomach, breast, lower bowel, cervix, mouth, lymphatic system, liver, throat, and prostate gland (*see box*). It is because this order seems to be reflected in most Western countries, where cancer is more common generally than in less developed countries, that cancer has been called 'a disease of civilization'.

---

**The ten commonest cancers**

| Worldwide | In America and Britain |
|---|---|
| Lung cancer (12 per cent) | Lung cancer (14 per cent) |
| Stomach cancer (10 per cent) | Skin cancer (non-melanoma) (12 per cent) |
| Breast cancer (9 per cent) | Breast cancer (10 per cent) |
| Colon cancer (9 per cent) | Colon cancer (6 per cent) |
| Cervical cancer (6 per cent) | Prostate cancer (5 per cent) |
| Mouth cancer (6 per cent) | Bladder cancer (4 per cent) |
| Lymphoma (4 per cent) | Stomach cancer (4 per cent) |
| Liver cancer (4 per cent) | Cancer of the rectum (4 per cent) |
| Throat cancer (4 per cent) | Cancer of the pancreas (2 per cent) |
| Prostate cancer (4 per cent) | Lymphoma (2 per cent) |
| Other cancers (34 per cent) | Others (36 per cent ) |

**The commonest cancers**

Based on the above listings, the commonest cancers, with their usual symptoms, are:

*Lung cancer*

Cancer of the lung is by far the most common form of cancer in the Western world, and is usually incurable. Over the past 50 years it has become the leading cause of death from cancer in men – although the number of female deaths from lung cancer has increased 50 per cent over the past 50 years.

Growths can also appear in the space in the chest called the *mediastinum*, but these are rare.

*Symptoms*
Typical symptoms of lung cancer are persistent breathlessness and coughing. The person may lose his or her appetite, feel permanently tired, and run a temperature.

*Skin cancer*

Skin cancer is another of the commonest cancers in the Western world. White-skinned people are most vulnerable because dark-skinned people are protected by their skin pigmentation from the damage that strong sunlight can do. This is why skin cancer is commoner among white people in hot countries such as Australia and South Africa – though cases are rising in Europe and North America, possibly because of the obsession with 'getting a good tan' in recent years.

There are three main types of skin cancer. In order of how commonly they occur, they are:

● *basal cell carcinoma* (or 'rodent ulcer')
● *squamous cell carcinoma* (also a type of ulcer)
● *malignant melanoma* (a 'melanoma' is a tumour of the cells (*melanocytes*) that give skin its colour)

The first two types appear mainly on exposed areas of the face, neck and arms. Malignant melanomas are the least common but the most threatening. They appear on the body and look like dark moles. They usually ulcerate within two or three months and penetrate deeply into the body tissues.

## Breast cancer

Among women breast cancer is the most common form of cancer in the West and the leading cause of death from malignant disease. But though there is a high rate of breast cancer in North America and Northern Europe it is rare in Asia and parts of Africa. One in every ten women in America and Britain is likely to develop breast cancer at some time in her life, though it is more common after the age of 50.

### Symptoms
The first sign of breast cancer is usually a lump or other change in the appearance of the breast. More details of the signs and symptoms to look for, and how to examine your own breasts, are described in chapter 4.

## Colon and rectum cancer

Tumours in the colon and rectum are very common, and are the second largest cause of death from cancer in the West. The fact that cancer of the colon is rare in Africa, Asia and South America indicates an almost certain link with the modern Western diet and lifestyle. This type of cancer can run in families, and usually affects people over the age of 50.

### Symptoms
The symptoms are vague pain, constipation alternating with diarrhoea, and passing blood in the stools.

### Prostate cancer

This type of cancer comes third only to cancers of the lung and bowel as a cause of death among men in the Western world. In the US twice as many black men die from it as white men, and the number of deaths from cancer of the prostate has risen steadily over the past 50 years in the UK, the US, and Australia. Men over 65 are most at risk, possibly because of reduced sexual activity with age.

### Symptoms

Often there are no specific symptoms, though there may be difficulty in passing urine due to enlargement of the prostate gland. Pain in the back and pelvis can mean that the cancer has spread to the bones.

### Bladder cancer

Cancer of the bladder is now the fifth most common cancer among men in the West. In the US, it is estimated that 45,000 new cases of bladder cancer occur each year. (Men working with aniline dyes in the rubber industry are particularly at risk it seems.) It is also common among smokers: at least half of cases in men and a quarter in women are due to smoking. Frequent bladder infections can also lead to cancer.

### Symptoms

Urgency and frequency of passing urine, sometimes with blood, is a common symptom, and there may be pain in the back or loins.

### Stomach cancer

The number of deaths from cancer of the stomach have decreased over the last ten years in both America and Britain but they remain high in countries such as Japan, China and Chile. More men than women are affected, usually the better-off.

*Symptoms*
Loss of appetite, nausea and vague stomach pain.

### Cancer of the pancreas

Cancer of the pancreas is linked with heavy drinking as well as with diabetes and is on the increase in most countries.

*Symptoms*
Pain, loss of weight and sometimes jaundice.

### Cancer of the lymphatic system

Cancer of the lymphatic system, or 'lymphoma', is the only one of the common cancers that is not a carcinoma, or cancer of the epithelial tissue (*see page 5*).

The best-known cancer of the lymphatic system is *Hodgkin's disease*, which affects all the glands, often starting with those in the neck and moving on throughout the body. A virus called the *Epstein-Barr* virus (EBV) is believed to be the cause. (The same virus also causes glandular fever.)

Hodgkin's disease most often strikes people between the ages of 10 and 20, and 50 and 70. It occurs more frequently in men than in women and it is more common in Western countries than Far Eastern countries such as Japan.

A variation is 'non-Hodgkin's lymphoma' (NHL). Also caused by viruses, this cancer attacks mainly the elderly – though children are sometimes affected.

*Symptoms*
The symptoms of Hodgkin's disease are painless swelling of the glands in the neck and armpits, coupled with fever and night sweats, loss of weight, and in some cases itching skin.

The main symptom of non-Hodgkin's lymphoma is usually painless swelling of the glands in the neck.

Non-Hodgkin's lymphomas can also spread to all the glands in the body.

## *Cervical cancer*

The second commonest cancer in women, after breast cancer, is cancer of the *cervix* (the neck of the womb). Cervical cancer is extremely rare in nuns, leading many experts to believe there is a strong link between the disease and having sexual intercourse with a number of partners. Women who are sexually active before the age of 20 are more likely to develop cancer of the cervix than women who become active later. Another possible cause is the herpes virus.

### *Symptoms*
Vaginal bleeding and an unpleasant discharge, often after intercourse.


## Less common cancers

Though cancer is possible in any part or organ of the body it is far less common in the following areas.

### *Head and neck*

Statistically, cancers of the head and neck affect men more often than women (the theory is that this is because men smoke and drink more). The throat is most susceptible, followed by the mouth and lips.

### *Throat*
Twice as many men as women get cancer of the throat (or *oesophagus*), usually between the ages of 60 and 80 (probably as a result of heavy smoking and drinking – though it could also be due to malnutrition). In the US it is more common among blacks than whites, and in poorer sections of society than in the better-off. It is also more common in France, Switzerland and South Africa than in the UK.

An early symptom of cancer of the throat is persistent hoarseness. Other common symptoms are difficulty in swallowing and loss of weight.

### Other cancers of the head and neck

Cancers inside the mouth may develop from mouth ulcers or sore places caused by ill-fitting dentures or accidental bites by sharp, jagged teeth. Cancer of the lip is a form of skin cancer and is often seen in elderly men. The ears, eyes and eyelids can be affected by cancer but such tumours are rare.

There are a number of glands in the head and neck vulnerable to tumours, including the salivary and thyroid glands, but these tumours are usually benign.

### Liver and gall bladder

### Cancer of the liver

This often follows cirrhosis of the liver. Again, men are more likely to get it than women, especially if they are over 50 and have suffered from cirrhosis of the liver for many years.

The liver is often affected as 'secondary' by primary cancers in other parts of the body.

### Cancer of the gall bladder

This may develop from liver fluke (a parasitic worm common in Africa) or gallstones and it is commonest in men and women over 65. Ulcerative colitis (an inflammation of the large bowel resulting in constant bloody diarrhoea and stomach ache) can lead to cancer of the colon. Symptoms are the same as for gallstones – pain, nausea, vomiting and jaundice.

### Small intestine

Although the small intestine, or bowel, represents three-quarters of the length of the whole digestive tract, cancer is rarely found there.

### Anus

Cancer in the anus is more common in women and male homosexuals. Symptoms are similar to piles (*haemorrhoids*), with pain and bleeding.

### Genito-urinary tract

The urinary tract (the kidneys, bladder and *urethra*) is the means of getting rid of liquid waste from the body (urine) and is very similar in men and women.

#### Cancer of the kidney

This is not common but very hard to treat if it does occur because diagnosis is seldom early. Symptoms are blood in the urine and pain in the kidney area.

#### Cancer of the ureter

The ureter is the tube that carries urine from the kidney to the bladder. Cancer here is also rare but symptoms are similar as for bladder cancer so making it hard to diagnose (*see page 10*).

### The male genitals

Apart from the prostate gland, the other common cancer of the male genitals is cancer of the testicles. Tumours rarely appear in the penis.

Men between the ages of 25 and 35 seem to be most vulnerable to cancer of the testicles, the incidence of which is steadily rising. Some 5,000 new cases are diagnosed in the US every year, and 800 in Britain. Symptoms are enlargement or lumps in testicles (*see* chapter 4).

### The female genitals

Apart from the cervix, the most common form of genital cancer found in women, cancer can sometimes also attack the lining of the womb (or *endometrium*), and the ovaries. It very rarely occurs in the vagina or vulva.

*Endometrial cancer*

Women between the ages of 50 and 70 are the usual victims of cancer of the lining of the womb. Cancers here grow very slowly and don't often spread, so they are rarely fatal. The risk factors are being overweight and the long-term (more than 3–4 years) taking of the drug Tamoxifen, which can be prescribed for breast cancer. The main symptom is bleeding from the vagina after the menopause.

*Ovarian cancer*

Though cancer of the ovaries is fairly common among women in Western countries it is more common among women who have had no children or who cannot have them. It can occur at the same time as breast cancer so some experts think it may be because of the same inherited tendency.

Symptoms of ovarian cancer are vague, making it difficult to diagnose at an early stage – so the disease is usually advanced by the time it is discovered.

*The nervous system*

Cancers of the nervous system are tumours of the brain, spinal cord and nerves. Tumours of the nerves, particularly the nerves furthest from the brain and spinal cord (*peripheral nerves*), are rare, as is cancer of the spinal cord. The most common are brain tumours.

*Brain cancer*

Brain cancer can cause the sufferer to become progressively more disabled and is very difficult to diagnose and treat. Brain tumours most often seem to happen in the first ten years of life, and between the ages of 50 and 60. Sadly, cases seem to be on the increase. In Britain, for example, where the disease caused 2,605 deaths in 1989, the incidence has risen nearly 24 per cent in just three years.

## *Cancer of the bones and soft tissue*

There are many different kinds of bone tumour, affecting both children and adults, but they are relatively rare. Tumours in the muscles and tendons (soft tissue) are extremely rare.

## *Cancer of the blood and bone marrow*

Leukaemia is the most familiar cancer of the blood and bone marrow (where most blood in the body is made). The disease causes the blood's white cells to proliferate and outnumber the red cells. The result is acute *anaemia*, a deficiency of red blood cells that makes the sufferer more likely to bleed and catch infections. Leukaemia most often attacks children under 18 and old people. Typical symptoms are fever, pain in the bones and joints, and swollen glands.

## Summary

The fact that the most common cancers among both sexes involve the lungs, digestive and urinary systems seems to point a very clear finger at modern diet, pollution and smoking as the likeliest causes of the rising number of cancer cases in the Western world.

With cancer, the lesson is to try and prevent it as far as possible and if not to start treatment early. The rest of this book looks at both strategies after explaining a bit more, in the next two chapters, about how and why cancer develops in the first place.

# CHAPTER 2

# Cancer and the immune system

*How and why cancer starts*

The key to cancer is the cell. The cell is the basic unit of life. Our bodies are made up of millions of cells that grow, reproduce by dividing into two, and then either die or rest until they are ready to grow and reproduce themselves again. This is called the 'cell cycle'. Every minute 300 million cells die and are immediately replaced by other cells, so that the number of cells in the body remains the same throughout life.

As figure 1 shows, a cell is made up of a core or 'nucleus' that controls and directs the cell's activities. The nucleus is contained inside a membrane and surrounded by a substance called 'cytoplasm'. This in turn is held within a porous membrane that allows various substances to move through in both directions: nutrients pass in and waste products pass out.

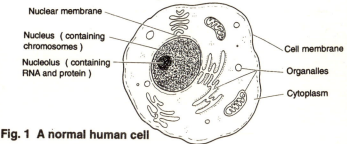

Nuclear membrane

Nucleus ( containing chromosomes )

Nucleolus ( containing RNA and protein )

Cell membrane

Organalles

Cytoplasm

**Fig. 1 A normal human cell**

Each cell has a particular job to do in keeping body tissues growing normally. Most important of all, the cells
must all work together in harmony if the body is to work
properly and stay healthy. Sometimes, though, for reasons not yet really understood, a single cell will run
amok. It breaks out of the normal cell cycle and starts
producing too many new cells. They in their turn start
reproducing, and this multiplication of cells forms an
abnormal growth (*see* figure 2).

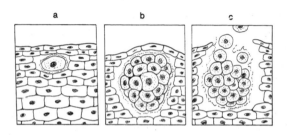

**Fig. 2  How cancer cells grow**

**How abnormal cells grow**

As explained in chapter 1, there are two kinds of abnormal cell growth: 'benign' and 'malignant'. What makes
one growth benign and another cancerous is not yet
known but both sorts of growth are the result of what is
called 'cell mutation'.

Mutation is possible in the human body at any time.
This means we all have the potential to develop cancer
at any time. What stops mutation is the body's own
built-in 'genetic coding'. Each of us has this coding in
every living cell. It is held and triggered by very special
chemicals called *DNA* (*deoxyribonucleic acid*) and *RNA*
(*ribonucleic acid*).

DNA holds all the information about a cell and is the

way a cell passes information on to its descendants while RNA is responsible for transferring the information and controlling its transfer. DNA and RNA together hold what we call our genetic coding or 'genes'.

Normally genes do not let anything interfere with them so that the same information is passed on in the same way to all future genes – thus making sure the plant or animal the cell is part of stays more or less the same. But sometimes, for various reasons, the system goes wrong.

Almost from out of nowhere, it seems, a 'blip' comes along that puts an error into the system and changes it. (Mutation actually means 'change in the genes of a cell'.) Most of the time in most people the body's own repair and maintenance system – more correctly known as 'the immune system' – is quick to spot and correct any error. But sometimes it slips up and an error goes unnoticed, resulting in a mutant gene being produced.

The mutant gene will start to divide like any other gene. If it survives beyond five or six 'cell cycles' it forms an abnormal or 'precancerous' cell. At this stage a strong immune system can still destroy abnormal cells if it wakes up to what is happening in time – and in most cases this is exactly what happens and why cancer is not as widespread as the common cold.

But if the immune system, for whatever reason, either does not respond or is not powerful enough to destroy the mutation then the cells start to grow strongly. They reproduce rapidly, changing their characteristics as they grow. This is what is called the 'promotion stage' and it is a critical phase in cancer cell growth. Some cancers do not get beyond it. Even now they can fail to establish themselves and die off.

Cancer cells that get beyond the promotion stage enter the 'progression stage' and this is when the disease really starts. At this stage the cancer is large enough to have developed its own blood supply and its own defence system and is developing into a full-blown, runaway growth. If the cancer is not stopped or removed at this point it simply continues to grow and spread until it overwhelms the healthy systems in the body, eventually causing death.


## The 'free radical' theory of cancer

The most convincing explanation to date of why cells go wrong is the action of what are called 'free radicals'. Free radicals are single oxygen molecules 'hungry' to mate or merge with another molecule to become a pair. Free radicals are an essential part of the way the human body works and are, indeed, a part of the body's disease-fighting mechanism.

Free radicals, if they work properly, are supposed to help in the regular clear-out of harmful substances in the body. But this delicate operation can, and does, go wrong frequently. And when it does, free radicals, in the words of British biochemist Professor David Blake, become 'the most powerful toxin in the body and a powerful system of destruction'.

Free radicals that go 'bad' turn against the body instead of protecting it. What happens is that they attach themselves to healthy cells and effectively send them out of control by damaging their inner core or nucleus. Cells damaged in this way either run amok and grow out of control, which is what happens in cancer, or shut down entirely and die.

It is this process that has led some pioneer researchers to think that the fundamental cause of cancer is free radical damage. But what makes free radicals turn crooked in the first place? Again, the best we have is a theory but it is a strong one, and one that is becoming stronger. The cause is probably a combination of the many things that most people face from the world around them – diet, environmental pollution and stress being the likely leading culprits (*see* chapter 3).

## All about the immune system

There is an important link between cancer and the immune system. The immune system is the key to the body's fight against cancer. If the immune response, which is nature's way of fighting off unwelcome intruders, becomes weak for any reason it may allow cancer cells to grow without being able to control them.

For this reason cancer can be seen as a disease of the immune system – or, rather, a disease of a failure of the immune system. Cancer is not the only example of a disease resulting from a weak immune system but it is by far the most serious example of it. Anyone with a weak immune system is at risk from intruders of all sorts.

The immune system is one of the most important systems in the body. Its job is to recognize, attack and destroy any and all abnormal tissue and intruders, or *antigens* as they are known. Viruses, harmful bacteria, fungi and 'allergens' such as house mites, pollen and dust are all antigens. So are rogue cells.

In a healthy person the immune system quickly and efficiently overcomes any threat to the normal working of the body by mobilizing its own 'home guard'. This is made up of white blood cells and chemicals in the blood known as *antibodies*. Antibodies destroy antigens by effectively eating them up and digesting and disposing of them as waste through the body's normal disposal systems. But, like any system, it can go wrong.

Uncontrolled or chaotic cell growth – cancer – is a result of the immune system going wrong and not doing its job properly, either by failing to spot a problem such as a rogue cell or by being too weak to do anything.

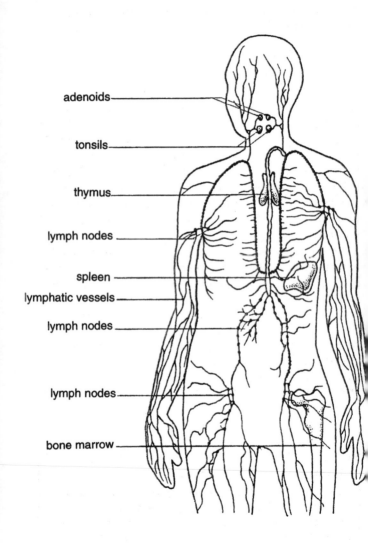

**Fig. 3 The immune system**

So understanding how the immune system works, and how it fights threats to the body, is important in treating cancer.

## How the immune system works

The immune system consists of your blood supply and lymphatic system. Both work together closely in the fight against disease. As figure 3 shows, the lymphatic system consists of a network of small channels running throughout your body (rather like blood vessels but carrying a fluid known as *lymph* rather than blood). These channels are connected to the circulatory system and three small sets of organs called the *thymus gland*, *lymph nodes* and the *spleen*.

Defence against disease is essentially a function of the 'white cells' in blood. White cells, known as *leukocytes.*, are made by the glands of the lymph system. Some white cells are also made in bone marrow (*see box*).

White blood cells produce the *antibodies* that defend the body against antigens. Antibodies are made by particular sorts of white blood cells known as *lymphocytes* and they come in five types, called *immunoglobins*:

---

**How blood fights infection**

The blood in our body is made up of roughly:

- 40 per cent red cells (known as *erythrocytes*)
- 60 per cent plasma, a semi-clear mixture of proteins (including vitamins) and mineral salts

A very small amount is made up of white cells (*leukocytes*) and special clotting agents called *platelets*. Other ingredients include the *hormones* that are the body's vital 'chemical controllers', controlling the body's essential activities.

---

Blood is made mainly in bone marrow (especially the long bones, the ribs, backbone, breastbone and skull) but also in the lymph nodes and spleen.

All red blood cells and some white cells come from bone marrow but white cells are also produced by the lymph nodes and the spleen.

White cells (leukocytes) come in three main types:

- *macrophages*
- bone-marrow cells (known as *B-cells*)
- thymus cells (*T-cells*)

Macrophages are large cells (seen through a miscroscope they are a mixture of round and elongated shapes) and are the major fighting cells. They are the 'cleaners-up'. They surround and 'hoover up' not only any harmful substance (antigen) such as a virus (*see* figure 4) but also the defending substance (antibody) before disposing of everything through the lymphatic system.

B-cells make antibodies that destroy antigens. They have a memory of past antigens.

T-cells are split into 'T-helpers', 'T-killers' and 'T-suppressors' and all are needed to keep the immune response balanced. T-killer cells contain *cytotoxins* that kill infected and cancerous cells and make an antigen-blocking protein called *interferon*.

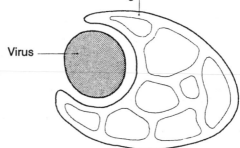

A macrophage (scavenger white blood cell) starts to engulf a virus

Virus

**Fig. 4 How blood attacks an antigen**

## How the immune system deals with an attack

The first thing that happens when an invader such as a virus or rogue cell is spotted by the immune system is that it makes a protein called *interferon*. This acts as a signal to other cells to resist the invader and stop it from multiplying.

Next the fighter T- and B-cells go into action. The blood supply to the digestive system slows down – which is why we often don't feel like eating – and our temperature rises. (A high temperature, or fever, is really a good sign. It shows the body is fighting back.)

T-cells fight antigens directly. They circulate around the body, passing on information about the invader and encouraging other cells to fight as well. B-cells make antibodies when they have the right information about the invader. This does not happen instantly, though. The immune system has to gather its forces to give good protection, and this gives the invader a little time to take hold – which is why symptoms of an infection often increase at first. The immune system has not had time to manufacture the new antibodies for the specific antigen attacking.

The bonus is that once the body has learnt to recognize the invader it does not need to repeat the manufacturing process in future. The next time the particular antigen tries to take over it will be recognized immediately and the defences swing into action without delay.

The particular problem for the immune system is that not everything coming into the body is bad for it. Some things, such as food and oxygen, are essential. So it must be able to tell the difference between the 'bad guys' and the 'good guys'. Fortunately nature has given the immune system a built-in programme that allows it to know what's good and what's bad. It is still constantly on guard, but because of this programming it will only attack those things in the body it sees as 'hostile', whether in the body such as abnormal cells (as in cancer) or coming into it from outside (such as bacteria and viruses).

Most of the time this system works fine but occasionally it fails. It most often fails because of the strength of the attack or because it has been weakened in some way and can no longer cope. It is when this happens that we become susceptible to illness of all kinds, including cancer.

## Summary

Cancer is abnormal cell growth or mutation, possibly due to free radical damage. But it is also the result of the failure of our immune system to work properly. So the clue to the cause of cancer lies in identifying those factors that not only make cells go berserk but also weaken the immune system.

The next chapter identifies the few known and the many suspected causes of cancer.

# CHAPTER 3

# Causes of cancer

*Known and suspected triggers and risk factors*

Research has been going on for many years to find out why cells should suddenly start forming abnormal growths, and a number of definite causes and triggers have already been discovered. But in many cases the cause is still unknown and various experts have a variety of explanations, some more accepted than others.

Certain cancers are known to be caused by a virus (liver cancer, a leading cause of death in Africa, is an example) but generally speaking cancer does not seem to be something you catch like flu or inherit from your parents. There is general agreement among most leading experts now that cancer is, like heart disease, very much a disease of poor lifestyle. It develops mostly for reasons of how you behave and the conditions you live in.

British scientists Sir Richard Doll and Richard Peto concluded after a review of causes of cancer in America in 1981 that three out of every four cancer deaths were the result of not living in a way that gives the body the support it needs to stay healthy.

Put simply that means cancer is predominantly a disease of not eating the right foods, drinking the right liquids, breathing the right air, thinking the right thoughts and taking the right exercise.

Cancer, like heart disease, has been called a 'disease of civilization'. Unlike heart disease, cancer was known in ancient times but cancer, like heart disease, is far more common in affluent developed countries with high levels of pollution than in cleaner, simpler societies.

A summary of known and suspected causes of cancer worldwide is very similar to that for heart disease: poor diet, mental and emotional distress, tobacco smoke, environmental pollution, alcohol, lack of exercise, infections and inflammation, and, sad to say, medical treatment.

How these causes relate to specific cancers is summarized in the table on page 33 but they can be grouped under five main headings. Not in order of importance these are:

- psychological distress
- food and diet
- chemical pollutants
- radiation
- infections and inflammation

Broadly speaking, the last four can all be classified as physical causes and there is relatively little argument about them as a result. The first, however, covering the psychological causes of cancer, is far more controversial.

## Psychological causes of cancer

The idea that the mind and emotions can influence health is extremely controversial in many conventional medical circles. The reason is partly to do with the fact that the way an individual's psychological makeup (that is, their mind and emotions) affects their health is harder to measure than the effect of physical factors such as diet or pollution.

But, again, the evidence, particularly from work in America, is that psychological factors can and do have a major impact on a person's physical state of health, influencing and even directly causing a wide range of diseases – including cancer.

In 1995 the pioneering Bristol Cancer Help Centre in south-west England added a second database to its one on diet (see 'Food and diet' on page 40), this time drawing together every piece of research showing the links between mind and emotions and cancer. Some 3,000 studies and 350 books published since the 1950s had been identified by the end of 1995 and from these the mind–body cancer link appears to be very strong.

A number of psychologists and psychotherapists, particularly in America, have even proposed the idea of a 'cancer personality' as a result of this link. In other words, some people are more prone to cancer because of the way they think and feel about themselves.

US therapist Debbie Shapiro, for example, author of *The Bodymind Workbook*, has described the cancer personality as one that is 'very loving, supportive and kind but simultaneously represses personal feelings, is long-suffering and with low self-esteem.' Cancer, she maintains, appears to be 'the result of many years of inner conflict, guilt, hurt, grief, resentment, confusion or tension surrounding deeply personal issues. It is connected to feelings of hopelessness, inadequacy and self-rejection. It has even been called "acceptable suicide".'

Research in the 1980s lent some support to this idea. For example, a British researcher, Dr Steven Greer of King's College Hospital in London, claimed to have found a close connection between survival of women with breast cancer and women who suppress negative emotions, especially of anger and anxiety. A number of other studies also found that women who did best against breast cancer were those who maintained a 'fighting spirit' while those who did worst were those with a helpless and hopeless attitude.

The latest thinking is very much against this idea of 'blaming the victim' and making them think it is somehow their fault if they get cancer but the basic idea that deeply rooted psychological factors play a part in the disease is now becoming more widely accepted.

The Bristol database, for example, shows, according to the centre's medical director Dr Rosy Daniel, 'clear evidence in support of the view that many of the common cancers have some of their origins in psychological factors'. These factors may depend on how particularly stressful experiences such as bereavement, divorce, being made redundant or fired, loneliness, isolation, lack of love and support affect the human spirit as well as more general psychosocial conditions such as religion, cultural background and attitude to life.

### Food and dietary causes of cancer

In 1994, the Bristol Cancer Help Centre compiled the largest database of research into the links between cancer and diet ever produced. Including more than 5,500 studies published in reputable journals since 1983, it supports the now widely held view that as many as 35 per cent of cancers may be diet related.

The link between food and disease of any sort, never mind cancer, is still controversial in conventional medical circles but even the most conservative researchers are now admitting that up to a third of cancers are probably diet related.

For example, a study in China published in 1993 showed that supplementing a diet low in essential nutrients with vitamins and minerals brought down cancer deaths by 13 per cent. Another study in Britain, published in the *British Medical Journal* in 1994, showed that vegetarians were 40 per cent less likely to die of cancer than meat-eaters.

## Chemical causes of cancer

As long ago as 1775 an English surgeon called Sir Percival Pott reported that a large number of chimney sweeps had skin cancer. The cause could only have been contact with soot. However, it was not until a century later that the penny began to drop when workers in the shale industry in Scotland, cotton-spinners in Lancashire, and people working in dye factories throughout the Western world developed a variety of cancers, mainly of the skin, lungs, colon and bladder.

These are the earliest modern examples of chemicals causing cancer – a process known as *chemical carcinogenesis* (any substance causing cancer is called a *carcinogen*). But since then, and particularly in the 20th century, the number of carcinogens in routine use has risen rapidly, contributing widely to the pollution of the air we breathe, the food we eat and the water we drink.

The main chemical carcinogens are:

- polycyclic hydrocarbons
- aniline
- dioxin
- aflatoxin
- alkylating agents

*Polycyclic hydrocarbons*
These are chemicals produced by burning anything containing carbon, and are present in coal-tar (from soot), tobacco smoke, car exhaust fumes, and some cooked (especially barbecued) meats. They are even in wood smoke. Polycyclic hydrocarbons are the most common and most serious chemical carcinogens.

*Aniline*
Aniline is an oily liquid made from coal tar and indigo, and is the raw material from which dyes are made. It has been known to cause cancer for more than a century but

is still in use. A new generation of dyes, known as *azo* dyes (used to colour foods like margarine yellow), have been developed but these are known to cause cancer too.

### Dioxin

Dioxin is a by-product of the chemical manufacturing industry. The process of bleaching paper also produces dioxin and burning plastic and rubber can give off dioxin as a gas. It is deadly and even small amounts can cause cancer. Large amounts kill.

### Aflatoxin

A chemical produced by the poisonous mould *aspergillus flavus*, which can contaminate foods stored too long. Aflatoxin can cause liver cancer.

### Alkylating agents

These are a group of drugs used to treat cancer and are an example of the treatment being worse than the disease. They destroy cancer cells – but can kill normal cells (usually white blood cells) at the same time, causing leukaemia.

### Other cancer-causing substances

Chemical substances that can cause cancer by being inhaled include asbestos, arsenic (in sheep dips), formaldehyde (a preservative used in plastics, pressed timbers and the plastic foam used in home insulation), and dust from coal, wood, brick, sand, fibre-glass or fibre-wool and metals such as aluminium, nickel and chromium.

Another cause of cancer by inhalation is radon, a natural radioactive gas that comes mainly from granite rock. Parts of Britain where granite is common such as Cornwall and Derbyshire are particularly badly affected. It can mount up underneath buildings built on granite and accumulate to dangerous levels. It is a cause of lung cancer if inhaled over a long period. Gas levels over 200 becquerels per cubic metre are serious and should be seen to.

A number of chemicals used in plastics, glues and paints are suspected of being carcinogenic and of causing both lung cancer and leukaemia. Nitrates, used in agriculture as fertilizers, and organochlorines, used in pesticides, may also cause stomach and throat cancer. Another suspect is fluoride added to water supplies to prevent tooth decay but, again, there is no definite proof of this.

## Summary of main cancer-causing substances

| Chemical | Cancer caused |
| --- | --- |
| Aflatoxin | Liver cancer |
| Aniline/azo dyes and derivatives | Bladder cancer, leukaemia |
| Asbestos | Lung cancer |
| Arsenic | Lung and skin cancer |
| Chromium, cadmium | Lung cancer |
| Crude oil | Leukaemia |
| Dioxin | Various cancers |
| Nickel | Lung and nasal cancer |
| Polyvinylchloride | Liver cancer |
| Polycyclic hydrocarbons | Lung, mouth and throat cancer |
| Radon | Lung cancer, leukaemia |

**Radiation as a cause of cancer**

Two main types of radiation are known to cause cancer:

● ultraviolet radiation, from the rays of the sun or a sun-lamp
● ionizing radiation, used in X-rays and in radiotherapy

But there is now growing evidence that a third category, radiation produced by electrically generated electromagnetic force fields such as those around overhead power lines, computers, microwave ovens, radar and modern telecommunications systems, may also trigger cancer.

## Ultraviolet radiation

In large doses ultraviolet radiation can cause skin cancer. 'Ultraviolet' means beyond the violet end of the spectrum, so ultraviolet rays can't be seen. In normal conditions they are absorbed by the ozone layer in the earth's atmosphere but in recent years damage to the ozone layer (largely from manmade environmental pollutants) has reduced the filtering effect of the layer and this has led, in turn, to dangerous levels of rays reaching the earth's surface.

## Ionizing radiation

Ionizing radiation is produced by radioactive material that has enough energy to knock electrons out of atoms to produce electrically charged atoms or 'ions'. Because ionizing radiation can kill cancer cells it is used in radiotherapy to destroy malignant growths. But it has to be used with great care because it can cause cancer as well as cure it.

Its power to cause cancer was first discovered during the First World War when women painting luminous watch dials with paint containing radium got bone cancer from licking their paint brushes to a fine point. Workers operating the early X-ray equipment, before protective clothing was worn, developed skin cancer for the same reason.

But it was its effects on the thousands of Japanese exposed to it when the first atomic bombs were dropped on Hiroshima and Nagasaki to end the Second World

War that brought it to public prominence. Nuclear power stations and the testing of nuclear bombs continue to risk today's population with a wide range of cancers.

X-rays can cause leukaemia, which is why their use in medicine is now a fraction of what it once was.

The maximum dose of radiation in a year should be 100 microsieverts. This compares with 20 microsieverts for the average chest X-ray, 50 microsieverts received by most people in Britain from Chernobyl nuclear power-station in 1986, and 5,000 microsieverts the nuclear industry is allowed to give its workers.

## Electromagnetic radiation

Modern electrical equipment produces a wide range of high and low frequency electromagnetic force fields (EMFs) and most people in the Western world are now facing 10,000 times the levels of half a century ago. Evidence is now building up that this exposure is by no means as safe and harmless as we would like to believe.

In 1992 Dr Dana Loomis of the University of North Carolina discovered that women working in the electrical industry suffered a 40 per cent higher death rate from breast cancer than other women. Studies since then, particularly in America, have shown a link between EMFs and both breast cancer and childhood leukaemia.

Background EMF radiation ranging between 60 and 120 nanotesla (nT) is normal in most modern buildings, but according to UK expert Simon Best 'some ten studies have now found an increased risk of childhood leukaemia in houses with EMFs as low as 200–300 nanotesla'.

Most recently, in 1995, the US National Council on Radiation Protection admitted a link between extremely low frequency (ELF) electric and magnetic fields and

Causes of the commonest cancers

| CANCERS | Lifestyle | | | | Environment/Occupation | | | | Infection |
|---|---|---|---|---|---|---|---|---|---|
| | Alcohol | Diet | Smoking | Sex | Stress | Pollution | Radiation | Sunshine | Viruses |
| Bladder | | | ● | | | | | | ● |
| Blood (leukaemia) | | | | | | | | | ● |
| Breast | | ● | | | ● | | ● | | |
| Cervical | | | | ●* | | | | | ● |
| Colon | | ● | | | | | | | |
| Liver | ● | ● | | | | | | | ● |
| Lung | | | ● | | | ● | ● | | |
| Lymph system | | | | | | | | | ● |
| Mouth | ● | ● | ● | ● | | | | | ● |
| Pancreas | ● | ● | | | ● | | | | ● |
| Prostate | | | | ●* | | | | | ● |
| Rectum | | ● | | ● | | | | | ● |
| Skin | | | | | | ● | ● | ● | |
| Stomach | | ● | | | ● | | | | |
| Throat | ● | ● | ● | | | | | | |

CAUSES & TRIGGERS

* Cervical cancer may be caused by too much sex too early while prostate cancer may be the result in older men of too little sex.

breast cancer and the American Environmental Protection Agency is to announce similar findings in 1996. ELF fields are created by equipment such as high-power lines, VDUs, microwave ovens, power lines and the latest telecommunications technology.

In Sweden EMF safety limits of 200 nanoteslas have already been proposed for all new schools and American authorities are considering following suit, mainly as a result of the suspected links between EMFs and cancer.

## Cancer caused by infection and inflammation

It was discovered early in the 20th century that animals might get cancer from viral infections, but it was not until the 1970s that it was found viruses could cause cancer in humans too. A notable example is the human immunodeficiency (HIV) virus that can lead to Aids: about 40 per cent of people with Aids develop a form of skin cancer called *Kaposi's sarcoma.*

Cancer of the cervix (the neck of the womb) can be caused by the herpes virus and, possibly, genital warts.

Another viral cause of cancer is the hepatitis-B virus, which can cause liver cancer. Hodgkin's disease (a cancer of the lymphatic system) and leukaemia (blood cancer) can result from viral infections too.

## Other causes

A variety of other factors may lead to cancer but cases are rare. The main ones are:

- *Genetic causes* Some forms of cancer can run in families through a faulty gene being passed from one generation to other but this is uncommon. As few as five per cent of breast cancers are estimated to be inherited, for example.

- *Hormone-dependent cancers*   Hormone-dependent cancers depend on the supply of hormones to grow. The sex organs of adult men and women are controlled by hormones and so cancers of the breast and uterus in women, and the prostate gland and testicles in men, are said to be 'hormone-dependent'. There are also fears that synthetic hormones created as a by-product of plastics manufacturing may be triggering cancer. Know as Xenoestrogens, they have been identified in some public water supplies. They are also used in intensive farming as growth-stimulators.
- *Various*   Cancers can develop where the skin or mucous membrane has been irritated, badly infected over a long period or scarred (mouth ulcers caused by ill-fitting dentures can become malignant, for example, if they remain for more than three or four weeks). Some chronic diseases such as ulcerative colitis (an inflammation of the large bowel) and Paget's disease (a bone disease) may also, occasionally, develop into cancer.

# CHAPTER 4

# How to help yourself

*Self-help methods for preventing
and alleviating cancer*

Cancer is a serious disease and not one to be taken lightly or trifled with. In fact it is regarded as so serious by authorities in many countries that it is actually illegal to treat yourself for it or to let anyone else who is not a doctor do so. This has tended to produce a widespead culture of fear, in which cancer is seen as some sort of inhuman plague that only experts in white coats with test-tubes and syringes can do anything about.

The unfortunate part of this is that it has allowed huge misunderstandings about cancer and its treatment to take root. Cancer is serious, but it is curable and cure does not have to take place at the hands of a medical expert. Self-cure has happened (doctors call them 'spontaneous remissions') and there are also many examples of sufferers having been helped by practitioners who are not doctors – by practitioners of natural therapy in other words.

Before treatment, though, comes prevention. That is to say, cancer does not become a problem if it can be prevented from happening in the first place and the evidence is clear that cancer can be prevented. Various estimates are that between 85 and 95 per cent of all cancers are preventable. So anyone who considers themselves at risk of getting cancer, for whatever reason, will benefit from the advice and guidance in this chapter.

But the chapter goes further. It also describes important ways in which the individual can help promote their own recovery if they already have cancer. There is nothing about miracle cures – they do not exist – but there are suggestions for the best ways of regaining some control over the disease – all of it based on tried and tested methods of helping yourself. No matter what you may be told there are very many safe, gentle and effective things you can do for yourself. (More on what natural therapies can help is in chapters 6, 7 and 8.)

## Preventing cancer

The first steps in preventing cancer are the same as for any disease in a world in which our body's defences are under regular threat from the way we live and the environment around us. It is a matter of taking a good look at our lifestyle and, very often, of making fundamental changes to the way we live and think. This is not always easy, but it is frequently essential if we really want to live a long, healthy and happy life – without cancer.

The three most important steps in cancer self-help are to look at our:

● food and diet
● mental and emotional (or psychological) state
● lifestyle and environment

## Food and diet

Claims have been made that various special diets can stop the growth of tumours in their tracks, and even shrink them. But, even though the scientific evidence for these claims has not yet convinced the majority of doctors, everyone is now agreed that there is a link between diet and cancer.

Research is still under way about precisely which foods may cause it and which prevent it. But all reputable cancer organizations around the world now recommend a diet low in animal fat and sugar and high in fibre-rich fruit and vegetables as a protection against cancer (*see* box on page 42). Some authorities suggest that many of us consume too much protein and this may have a link with cancer also.

Examples of known or suspected links between food and cancer are:

- obesity and a high fat intake with breast cancer
- smoked and salted foods with stomach cancer
- charred meat or meat grilled over an open flame (as in a barbecue) with all forms of cancer, particularly bowel cancer

The fact there seems to be a definite connection between diet and bowel cancer, for example, is known because people in Africa who eat a high-fibre diet with plenty of rice in it seldom get it, while people in the West who eat more meat, butter and other fatty foods, frequently do.

The theory is that high-fibre foods form bulky waste matter that passes through the gut quite quickly, and this doesn't give toxins a chance to accumulate and start a malignancy. But, though eating a healthy and nutritious diet is one of the very best ways of not only preventing cancer but helping in the fight against it if you've got it, the story does not end there. The next step is to take in specific extra nutrients that actually fight disease.

---

**Guidelines for eating against cancer**

- Eat less fat (trim all the fat off meat, and try fish or chicken instead).
- Buy only skimmed or semi-skimmed milk, low-fat yoghurt and cheese.
- Cut down on fried food (bake, grill or steam it instead).
- Eat low-fat margarine (without hydrogenated fat) instead of butter; give up cream.
- Eat more fibre (or 'roughage'). That means eat
  - at least five portions of fresh fruit and vegetables every day (leave the skin on fruit but wash carefully)
  - dried fruit, especially prunes (without sugar)
  - plenty of dark green and yellow vegetables (spinach, broccoli, carrots)
  - baked potatoes with the skins left on
  - plenty of wholegrain cereals (eg brown rice)
  - muesli, bran flakes, or porridge for breakfast
  - wholemeal flour and wholemeal bread only
  - wholemeal pasta
- Eat less sugar. That means
  - cut down on cakes, biscuits, sweets and chocolate
  - eat fresh fruit for dessert instead of a pudding
- Eat less salt. That means
  - cut down the salt added in cooking and at table
  - cut out snacks like crisps and salted nuts
- Eat organic as far as possible.

---

*How food fights cancer*

As explained in chapter 2, an important part of the cancer story is free radical damage. As well as being a possible, or even probable cause of cancer, free radical damage is the reason we age. Ageing is the process of our bodies oxidizing and is exactly the same process as iron going rusty or butter going rancid.

Luckily, there is a natural antidote to free radical damage and it is in the form of specific chemicals in food known as vitamins and minerals. Vitamins such as A, C and E and minerals like selenium, zinc and manganese have a natural 'antioxidant' action – they act against the process of 'oxidization' that free radicals can cause. Naturally, they are called 'antioxidants'.

Foods that contain antioxidants are therefore a powerful protection against cancer. The most potent combination of food in the fight to prevent cancer are those that contain high amounts of vitamins A, C and E, the minerals selenium, zinc and manganese, and dietary fibre. The best sources of all these are as follows.

### Vitamin A

In its natural form of beta carotene, which the body converts to vitamin A, it is found in deep-yellow and orange fruit and vegetables such as apricots, oranges, peaches, melons, bananas, carrots, pepper and sweet potatoes. It is also found in dark green vegetables such as spinach, broccoli and spring greens.

### Vitamin C (or ascorbic acid)

This is contained in most citrus fruits (such as oranges, lemons, limes and grapefruit) and tropical fruits (guavas, kiwi fruit, pawpaws and mangoes) but other excellent sources are red and green peppers, Brussels sprouts, strawberries, tomatoes and potatoes. It is one of the few essential vitamins the human body cannot make for itself and so has to be taken in the diet or as a food supplement. Vitamin C is the most powerful antioxidant after vitamin E.

### Vitamin E

Vitamin E is the single most powerful antioxidant known. It is found particularly in unsaturated vegetable oils (such as soybean and sunflower seed oil) and nuts such as almonds, walnuts and cashews. Peas, beans and some leafy vegetables are also good sources.

*Selenium*

This mineral is found in many different foods, including meat (particularly liver and pork), fish and seafood (eg clams and shrimps), mushrooms, milk, eggs, vegetables such as onions, garlic, courgettes and cabbage, and wholegrain foods.

*Zinc*

Zinc deficiency is thought to be a factor in some cancers, particularly that of the prostate. It has been used in prevention and treatment and may strengthen the immune response. A study in Turkey found that prostate cancer patients had low zinc levels compared with those whose prostate enlargement was benign. Zinc is high in shellfish (it is exceptionally high in oysters) but it is also in fish, liver and eggs.

*Manganese*

Good sources of manganese are wheatgerm, cereals, brown rice and egg yolk.

*Dietary fibre*

This is the part of the foods we eat that cannot be digested and absorbed, so passes right through the digestive system and out at the other end. It is found in the husks on wheat and other cereal crops and the skin on fruit and vegetables. It adds to the bulk of the waste products, and makes the stools softer, so that they pass more quickly and easily out of the body. This is why fibre is such a good natural remedy for constipation.

### Food (or dietary) supplements

If your nutrient intake is not as high as you think it should be, or your exposure to pollutants is high and you would like to take extra amounts of those nutrients known to help prevent or combat cancer, you can take them in concentrated form as food supplements. Food,

or dietary, supplements come in the form of tablets, cap-
sules, powder and liquid. Taking them as a preventive
measure is a sensible thing for anyone to do who considers themselves at risk and the box below shows you the
amounts recommended by the Bristol Cancer Help
Centre in England to ward off cancer.

Treatment for cancer by supplements is a more serious matter and so should really only be done under the
guidance and supervision of a specialist in nutritional
medicine such as a nutritional therapist or naturopath
(*see* chapter 8). Some doctors understand how to use
supplements but not enough. Nutrition is still hardly
touched on at most medical schools so be wary of any
doctor who says supplements only give you 'expensive
urine' – the usual jibe.

---

**Supplements to prevent cancer**

| *Supplement* | *Dose* |
|---|---|
| Beta carotene (Vitamin A) | 1x6mg tablet twice a day |
| Vitamin B complex | 1x50mg tablet a day |
| Vitamin C (as calcium or magnesium ascorbate) | 1x500mg tablet three times a day |
| Vitamin E | 1x133mg tablet or 200iu a day |
| Selenium (optional) | 1x200mcg tablet a day |
| Fish oil and flaxseed (linseed) oil OR | 400–500mg a day |
| Evening primrose oil | 1500–2000mg a day |

*Note* In spite of some scaremongering food supplements
are perfectly safe if used according to makers' instructions.
Some supplements (such as vitamin A in its artificial form of
retinol, zinc and selenium) can be toxic but only if taken in
large amounts, far higher than any of the levels above. But
it is always best to double-check with someone who knows
what they are talking about when it comes to using
supplements therapeutically (*see* chapter 8).

---

## Psychological distress

Initially what we call 'stress' is a natural, bracing reaction to extra physical or mental demands and a certain amount of it is not only unavoidable but necessary and healthy. It keeps us alert and alive. But too much, as the American stress pioneer Dr Hans Selye showed, can tip us over the edge. It is when stress is never-ending that illness can result.

Of course there are plenty of events producing mental and emotional distress we can do little to control, such as problems at work or with the bank manager. But there are steps we can take to avoid or remove the effects of prolonged and repeated strain – all of which can undermine the body's ability to adapt. Many of the techniques popular for reducing the strain of life in general are also now being used to help people combat illness of all sorts, including cancer.

For example, an excellent antidote for too much stress is exercise. That does not necessarily mean 'working out' in a gym or club but going swimming, or for a long walk or cycle ride. Exercise is an essential part of staying healthy but few people understand how good it is also at 'de-stressing'. So, if stress is a problem, the moral is – make time for exercise. It not only helps prevent cancer but can assist in treatment and recovery too.

Other anti-stress tips are to learn how to relax properly and to express feelings more spontaneously. Not relaxing and not expressing feelings are both risk factors in cancer, particularly for those used to bottling their feelings up and putting a brave face on hardship. If you already have cancer, what matters most is adopting a positive approach to fighting the disease. Most studies of 'fighting spirit' suggest that this improves patients' quality of life and survival chances.

All the following methods encourage the mind to help the body by adopting a positive approach to oneself and one's problems.

## For relaxation

'Movement' therapies such as yoga and t'ai chi are exceptionally good ways of learning to relax that anyone can learn for themselves very easily (*see* chapter 8 for more on these therapies).

Another effective self-help method is 'floating' – you float in a few inches of warm salt water inside an enclosed chamber or 'tank', preferably in the dark or with your eyes closed – and listening to relaxing music.

To 'float' you need to find a centre or clinic that offers this service but a simpler way of achieving the same effect is to soak in a hot bath with all the lights out and the blinds down to make it as dark as possible. Some people find that adding an essential oil like lavender to the water and burning a candle or two as they soak extra relaxing.

For those who would rather sit in an armchair and listen to relaxing tapes the British Holistic Medical Association publishes audio-tapes for relaxation as part of its *Tapes for Health* series, as does the Yoga Biomedical Trust in London and the Bristol Cancer Help Centre, also in Britain (*see* appendix *A* for details).

If you are one of those people who simply finds it impossible to stop and switch off, the best way of relaxing is probably to turn to the services of therapists who specialize in stress reduction such as massage therapists, aromatherapists and reflexologists. Of course a sympathetic and skilful partner could do just as well but professional help is likely to be more effective (*see* chapter 8).

**A simple relaxation exercise**

The following exercise is often taught as a part of relaxation therapy and is found very valuable by many people. Once learnt the technique is easy to practise at home. All you need is 20 minutes of peace and quiet, preferably in a room by yourself, where you can lie flat on the floor. The aim is to empty your mind of all negative thoughts, to visualize the beauties of a peaceful scene, and to imagine the sounds of nature that will bring that scene to life in your mind.

Having set your scene to achieve peace and tranquillity of mind, next begin to relax all your muscles, taking one group at a time. Start with your toes and feet, continue with your fingers and hands, first contracting and then relaxing a muscle group so that eventually all your limbs feel heavy and inert. If someone lifted one of your arms it would just flop back on the floor.

Continue the process of contracting and relaxing muscle groups all the way up the body, even to your eyebrows and scalp, and when you are completely relaxed just lie there for a while as if letting your body sink through the floor. Then bring yourself back to reality slowly and gently, without any hurry. You will be amazed how much calmer and more in control you feel when you get up.

Relaxation exercises can be coupled with deep-breathing exercises, which are also good for helping you to release tension. Physical therapists teach both breathing exercises and relaxation techniques, and you should have no trouble in finding one who is well qualified.

*For 'letting go' and being positive*

There are a number of specialist therapies that can help someone with real difficulty in this area. Examples are counselling, psychotherapy, hypnotherapy, and 'art' therapies such as music, dance, art and drama therapy, but all must be done through a properly trained and qualified practitioner for real benefit (*see* chapter 7).

Among tried and tested techniques that, once learnt, anyone can do for themselves are meditation and visualisation. For more on these, *see* chapter 7.

## Lifestyle and environment

It is unavoidable and clearly impossible to be able to control our surroundings completely but there are many things we can control. For example, we can control the circumstances we put ourselves in deliberately and what we do when we're in them. Examples of 'avoidable pollution', all leading causes of cancer, are:

- smoking
- drinking
- sunbathing
- unsafe sex
- working in dangerous surroundings at home or work

### Smoking

All cancer specialists agree that inhaling tobacco smoke – which contains coal tar – is at least as big a cause of cancer as diet. It causes not only cancer of the lung, but also of the throat, the kidneys, the pancreas and the bladder, all of which are difficult to treat and may be fatal.

Tobacco smoke is not only dangerous to those who smoke cigarettes or pipes, but also to non-smokers who breathe in their smoke. This is known as 'passive smoking', and it carries risks of making chest diseases such as asthma and bronchitis worse, as well as provoking cancer. It's also worth remembering that smoking is a leading cause of heart disease, which kills more people even than cancer.

One eminent British cancer specialist, Sir Richard Doll, carried out research into the effects of giving up smoking with a group of doctors who were all smokers.

After 12 years of total abstinence from cigarettes, the risk of the doctors developing lung cancer had fallen to the same level as non-smokers. The risk was considerably reduced even in those who had been exceptionally heavy smokers.

So the moral here is clearly to cut out smoking altogether if you can, or reduce it to a minimum if you can't.

### Drinking

Smoking and drinking often go together, and are common social habits throughout the modern world. They obviously give much pleasure but they can also cause cancer of the mouth and throat. Too much alcohol can also lead to cancer of the liver and pancreas (usually after causing *cirrhosis* of the liver first).

The moral here, again, is moderation: cut your intake of alcohol down to a level where it will still give you pleasure but do you no harm. Doctors disagree about what exactly safe limits are for healthy people but most experts think about three to four units a day is safe for men and two to three for women. A unit is a glass of wine, a shot of spirit or a small glass of beer. But alcohol is best avoided for those with cancer if possible.

### Sunbathing

Cancers of the skin, frequently caused by the ultraviolet rays of the sun, are now so common among white-skinned people that it is essential to be particularly careful how, when and where you expose yourself to sunshine, particularly if you have a fair skin that freckles and burns easily.

Many people, especially those on holiday in hot countries, either don't realize or forget that the sun's rays are strongest between 11am and 3pm – and that they can damage the skin even through sunscreens and *even through cloud*.

**Case history**

Diplomat Robert, 35, never thought of himself as a sun-worshipper, although he loved windsurfing and his job frequently took him to hot countries where he could enjoy an outdoor life.

One day he noticed a mole on his back that was growing bigger, had begun to itch, then bleed, and become crusted. After six weeks he went to see his doctor, who sent him for a biopsy of the mole. It proved to be a malignant melanoma, which was removed by surgery, leaving a long, unsightly scar on his back.

A year later another tumour appeared in his groin, which was also removed, together with the nearby glands. Robert then had to endure a two-year course of chemotherapy to prevent any more melanomas appearing.

Sunbathing should always be done in easy stages using sunscreens. But sunscreens are not a protection against skin cancer in spite of advertising that says they are. In fact some experts think they may even increase the risk by giving a false sense of security. The lesson here is always, but always, cover up, wearing a hat and long-sleeved clothing, when the sun is at its height.

### Unsafe sex

Herpes, a virus that can be passed from one sexual partner to another, is linked to cervical cancer as are genital warts – also passed on through sex. So there is the same case for moderation in sexual activity as in drinking and sunbathing.

Ironically, lack of sex has been suggested as a reason

for prostate cancer in older men. The gland may have become cancerous because of its under-use by men as they have got older.

## Hazardous surroundings at home or work

You are definitely at risk of cancer if you are routinely surrounded by industrial dust and other substances, and probably at risk if constantly subject to electromagnetic fields from appliances such as computers and microwave ovens, though experts are still arguing about this (*see* chapter 3).

Protect yourself from dangerous dust by always wearing a face mask and protective clothing or by following safety advice (where it exists). If no advice exists play safe and take precautions anyway. Laws in most responsible countries oblige employers to meet strict health and safety standards in these situations and they should not only allow you to follow the rules but insist on it. Have no hesitation in reporting any that don't.

It is not as easy to avoid inhaling exhaust fumes from road traffic, insecticides used in some crop sprays or the arsenic in sheep-dips, but public protest against this kind of pollution is strong and getting stronger, resulting in tighter controls. However, constant pressure needs to be kept up everywhere.

### Radiation pollution

The main dangers are from electrical appliances producing low-frequency electromagnetic radiation such as microwave ovens and computers.

● Make sure computer screens have a filter over them and do not sit or work close (within a metre) of a TV or computer screen or within two metres of the back or sides of another computer monitor, television screen or other form of visual display unit (VDU).

- Do not live or work close to high-voltage power-lines (the electromagnetic radiation fields extend several hundred yards).
- Always turn off electrical appliances, especially computers, when not needed.
- Make sure floors and inlets of buildings subject to radioactive radon gas from granite rocks are properly sealed and tested and have under-floor ventilation.
- Do not have unnecessary X-rays and if you do have one make sure the dentist or doctor puts a protective bib or shield over any part not being X-rayed (and have lots of iodine in your diet at the same time – for example, kelp tablets – as this helps to expel the radioactivity from your system).
- Avoid clocks and watches with luminous dials.

People who routinely live or work in surroundings with high levels of any form of radiation should have regular medical checks, including blood tests.

*Packaging pollutants*
Many packaging materials contain small amounts of cancer-causing substances that can get into food and drink, especially those based on plastic materials such as transparent film for wrapping up food, milk and juice cartons and plastic bottles. Use waxed paper or foil to wrap food and buy drinks in glass bottles. Store food in china, earthenware, glass or stainless-steel containers.

*Air pollution*
If you feel the air around you is polluted, especially outside, wear a face-mask or wrap a fine-weave scarf (such as silk) around your nose and mouth. Beware of inhaling smoke from fires, especially from burning plastic and rubber. Inside, never sit in a room of smokers or where there is a coal or wood fire without proper ventilation.

Avoid products with formaldehyde such as cavity-wall insulation and pressed timbers.

*Water pollution*
Using a good water filter is almost essential in most areas with a public water supply. Even natural spring sources are likely to have some pollution so filtering is still advisable. Let tap water run for a bit to clean out any collected impurities before drinking.

**Summary**

Self-help can make a big difference in the fight against cancer, particularly in preventing it in the first place (and especially in preventing it returning if you have already had successful treatment for it earlier).

However, there is no doubt that the very diagnosis of cancer is a catastrophic blow for many people and the need to see and talk to a sympathetic health professional is almost the most important part of any treatment. In the rest of this book we'll look at what health professionals of different sorts – both conventional and unconventional – offer those unfortunate enough to have been diagnosed as having cancer.

## Self-examination for men and women

Besides keeping an eye out for any of the common warning signs (*see* chapter 1), you can examine yourself more closely for the symptoms of the most common types of cancer: cancer of the breast, testicles, skin and bowels.

### Checking your breasts

Becoming 'breast aware' – becoming really familiar with the normal shape and feel of breasts and looking and feeling regularly for any changes – is now official health policy for women in most Western countries. The sort of unusual changes, or abnormalities, to look for are:

- any small lump or swelling in the breast or armpit
- any unusual increase in the size of one breast
- a dimple or dent in the skin when lifting the arm
- any reddish, ulcerated or scaly area of skin on the breast or nipple
- any bleeding from the nipple, or moist, reddish areas that don't heal easily
- any change in the position of the nipple – that is, pulled inward or pointing up or down
- any rash on or around the nipple
- a change in the colour of the skin
- veins showing up more than normal

Some organizations specializing in information and advice about cancer encourage women to examine their breasts at a fixed time each month. A good time is at the end of a period (if you are still menstruating). Breasts are less likely to be normally lumpy or tender at this time. Women who no longer have periods could check their breasts on the first day of each month. If you do discover a lump, report it to your doctor right away, remembering that by no means all lumps in the breast are malignant. But one that is should be diagnosed and removed as quickly as possible to give treatment the best chance of success.

### How to do it

Stand in front of a mirror and change the position of your

arms so that the breasts also change position. Next, lie down on a flat surface with a pillow under your head and a folded towel under one shoulder to raise it slightly. The flat of the fingertips of the opposite hand should be used to examine the raised breast.

### Checking your testicles

It is important for men, particularly young men, to check their testicles regularly. Testicular cancer attacks men between the ages of 25 and 35, but it is curable if it is caught early enough. It usually attacks one testicle, although both may be affected.

The early signs are a painless swelling or lump in the testicle, a heavy feeling in the scrotum (the pouch that contains the testicles), or a dull ache in the groin or the pit of the stomach. All young men should check their testicles once a month. It is less trouble to do while in a warm bath or having a shower, when the skin of the scrotum will be relaxed and easy to handle.

### How to do it

Start by supporting the scrotum in the palm of one hand, and note the size and weight of the testicles. It is perfectly normal for one to be larger and heavier than the other. But it helps to know which one is larger and hangs lower so as not to be misled into thinking it is abnormal. Examine each testicle in turn, very gently, using both hands to roll it between the fingers and thumbs to check for any lumps, unusual swellings, or hardness. It's a good idea to get really familiar with how they feel. For instance, there is a long, cord-like structure lying at the back of the testicle, called the *epididymis*, which stores and transports sperms. This can get separated from the testicle when the scrotum is warm and relaxed, and could easily be mistaken for an abnormality.

### Checking your skin

Check your skin regularly for such tell-tale signs as spots, moles or ulcers that won't heal and continue to grow in size.

Basal cell and squamous cell skin cancers (*see* page 8) on the face, hands and arms are curable by conventional surgery and radiotherapy if they are diagnosed soon enough. Even malignant melanomas on the body can be treated successfully if caught in time. Report any of the following signs to your doctor as soon as you can:

- a mole that itches
- a mole that is bigger than the blunt end of a pencil
- a mole that keeps increasing in size
- a mole that has a ragged outline
- a mole that is brown and black instead of all one colour
- a mole that is inflamed, or has a reddish edge
- a mole that is bleeding, oozing, or crusting

### *Checking your bowels*

There are usually no outward signs of bowel cancer so the only real way of checking is to keep a close watch on your bowel habits. Any consistent change in them may be the first sign of a tumour.

One obvious sign of potential trouble is passing blood with your stools. Any symptom of this sort should be reported to your doctor immediately. Bleeding from the rectum can be caused by the very painful condition known as piles (*haemorrhoids*). These can be the result of straining to pass stools if you are constipated. They are not dangerous, and can be quite easily treated.

Bleeding in the bowel can also be caused by *polyps* (small benign growths) and these too can easily be removed. Polyps, though, can sometimes be what is called 'pre-malignant'. That is, they may be the very start of cancer – so the sooner they are detected, removed, and sent for analysis the better.

Another common sign is a change in your normal bowel habits. Everyone's habits are different but if your normal routine changes you should take note and let your doctor know. You should do this particularly if you become first constipated and then have diarrhoea, and this pattern continues.

# CHAPTER 5

# Conventional treatments for cancer

*What doctors and surgeons are likely to say and do*

As already explained, cancer is a malignant proliferation of cells that cannot be contained and keeps on growing. So conventional medicine aims to detect and remove or destroy these cells at the earliest possible stage, before they have time to move on from their original site and do mischief elsewhere, and prevent them from recurring.

Doctors know that cancer is by no means always fatal. Some types, such as testicular cancer, can be cured. The cure rates are now extremely high for this form of cancer by conventional methods: more than 80 per cent.

But doctors also know that all types of cancer, even very difficult ones to deal with such as lung cancer, have a much better chance of cure if they are detected at the earliest possible stage in their development.

So the attitude of most doctors is that if a cancer can be detected at the first stage of its development, while it is still localized and before it has started to spread, there is a good chance that it can be stopped in its tracks and the patient cured. Five years free of cancer is the magic figure as far as the medical profession is concerned, even though in reality the period is fairly abitrary.

Patients have to return to the centre where they have been treated for regular checks – first every three months, then every six, and then every year for five years. If, after five years, there is still no sign of the cancer returning doctors regard it as officially cured.

## Diagnosing cancer

All doctors know that recovery from cancer is most likely if the disease is caught early on. That means early diagnosis. Cancer, unfortunately, is one of those diseases in which symptoms often only really start to be felt after it has lodged itself for some time and is quite far advanced.

It is for this reason that most doctors support regular 'screening' programmes to catch cancer before it has a chance to 'take root' and so prevent it spreading. Examples of established screening programmes include, for women, the 'Pap smear test' for cervical cancer and mammography (X-ray of the breast) for breast cancer.

Similar tests have been proposed in some countries for men to check for signs of common cancers such as cancer of the prostate and testicles. But, in spite of support from doctors, public screening programmes are expensive and are under growing threat. This follows recent criticism from the accountants and politicians who run such services that they have not been proved to save lives and so may not be worth the cost.

In the absence of regular screening, the responsibility is on the individual to notice any change in their body as soon as it happens and report it to their doctor. A good doctor, knowing the importance of early diagnosis in cancer, should immediately refer anyone showing suspicious symptoms (*see* chapter 1) for one or all of the following tests:

- biopsy
- blood tests
- X-ray (and barium enemas)
- ultrasound scan
- CT (or 'Cat') scan
- nuclear imaging
- endoscopy

Because cancer is such a difficult and dangerous disease, and because conventional medicine has therefore devoted a high degree of specialization to it, the tests will almost always be done at a specialist department in a hospital or specialist clinic. The supervising doctor will be someone known as an *oncologist* – oncology being the conventional medical term for the study and treatment of tumours (so cancer centres are usually also known as *oncology* departments or clinics).

## Biopsy

A biopsy is the procedure of taking a small piece of tissue for analysis. With growths just under the skin it can be done by 'needle aspiration', either (without a local anaesthetic) using a very fine needle, or (under a local anaesthetic) with a larger needle, which is part of a device rather like a tiny apple-corer. The needle is inserted into the growth and withdraws (or aspirates) a tiny part of it for examination.

## Blood tests

A small amount of blood may be taken from a patient, through a needle, to check what doctors call the blood 'count' and the other chemical ingredients in the person's blood. A blood count gives the amount of red and white blood cells in blood. Since levels vary depending on disease and drugs given, a blood count is a very good indication not only if disease is present but the effect various drugs are having on it.

For this reason blood tests are frequently done after a course of treatment such as chemotherapy as well as beforehand for diagnostic purposes. Blood tests are also used in nutritional therapy to see if someone is deficient in specific nutrients.

## X-ray

In use for more than a century as a means of getting a picture of someone's insides without cutting them open, X-ray is used in cancer diagnosis mainly for detecting tumours of the lung or breast. There has been some concern recently that the squashing of breasts in breast X-ray (mammography) may spread existing cancer.

A development of straight X-raying, particularly in the diagnosis of bowel cancer, is the use of X-rays with the radio-opaque substance barium. The patient is fed barium in a meal (hence the term 'barium meal') or inserted up the back passage (hence 'barium enema') and then X-rayed. The barium outlines the gut and shows up any growth and this is shown on the X-ray.

## Scans

'CT' and 'Cat' are nicknames for *computerized tomography*, a diagnostic technique that marries X-ray with computer technology. A detailed picture of organs deep inside the body is built up by a computer from X-ray readings and displayed on the computer monitor. Unlike with X-rays, no film is necessary with this method.

## Ultrasound

Another non-invasive test to give the same picture of internal organs on a screen, ultrasound uses high frequency sound waves instead of X-rays. It is completely painless and, unlike X-rays, relatively safe but the reason it is not used more in cancer diagnosis is that doctors say it does not give an accurate enough picture of many forms of cancer. It is used mainly to detect cancers of the brain and urinary tract.

### Nuclear imaging

Two main sorts of nuclear imaging test are used in cancer diagnosis:

- *Magnetic resonance imaging (MRI)* is a new technique in which radio waves are beamed at the body while it is placed in a magnetic field 50,000 times stronger than the earth's magnetic field. Signals given off are converted into a picture by a computer. Again, no X-rays are used but the process is slow and expensive and the side-effects are not yet known.
- *Isotope scans* involve giving a patient a very small amount of a mildly radioactive substance such as iodine by injection (or in the case of the thyroid, by mouth) and scanning the tissues being investigated. The tissues take up the radioactive substance and give off rays that the scanner can detect. The method is particularly useful for pinpointing bone or liver cancers.

### Endoscopy

This is a technique using the very latest in fibre-optic technology and a piece of equipment known as an *endoscope*. This is a long, thin, flexible tube made of tightly-packed glass fibres through which light can be transmitted to the tip of the instrument. When it is inserted into the body the surgeon can see the inside of the organ being inspected through an eyepiece. Through another 'pipe' in the tube the surgeon can wash out the area he or she wants to look at in order to see it more clearly, and also take a small piece of tissue – or 'smear' – to be analysed in the laboratory.

The same type of instrument is used for looking at different parts of the body, but the name changes: a *bronchoscope* is used for the lungs, a *gastroscope* for the stomach, a *colonoscope* for the lower bowel or colon, and so on. The endoscope is usually inserted with a local anaesthetic so that there is no pain or discomfort, and the patient attends as an outpatient.

It is used particularly in the investigation of cancers of the bowel (when the endoscope is fed in through the anus) and stomach (when it is put in through the mouth).

## Treating cancer

Having established that a malignant growth is present most doctors will want to start treatment immediately – and that usually does mean immediately. Depending on the severity of the growth discovered treatment can begin literally within hours of a diagnosis being confirmed.

Conventional medicine generally relies on three main weapons in its treatment of cancer:

● surgery
● radiotherapy
● chemotherapy

Until the advent of modern 'scientific' medicine, surgery was the only treatment available. But this century surgery has been joined by, first, radiotherapy and, since the 1950s, by chemotherapy. Surgery is now part of a three-pronged attack in which it is used either on its own or in combination with radiotherapy and chemotherapy, according to the type of tumour to be treated.

## Summary of conventional treatment for common cancers

| Type of cancer | Treatment | Success rate |
|---|---|---|
| Lung | Surgery, radiotherapy | Poor. Usually lung cancer is too far advanced by the time it is diagnosed to treat with much hope of success |
| Breast | Surgery, chemotherapy | Good, but only if caught early. Cure is much more uncertain if the tumour has spread to the lymph nodes |
| Throat | Surgery, radiotherapy | Good, if caught early |
| Stomach | Surgery | Poor, mainly because of the difficulty of early diagnosis |
| Liver | Surgery | Good, but only if caught early and the tumour is small (the liver can renew itself even if three-quarters of it is removed) |
| Pancreas | Surgery, radio/chemotherapy | Poor |
| Gall-bladder | Surgery | Fair, if caught early |
| Colon | Surgery | Fair, if caught early |
| Anus | Radiotherapy | Good, 60 per cent survival after five years |
| Kidney | Surgery | Fair, if the tumour is small and has not spread (but the whole kidney must be removed. Some 25 per cent of kidney tumours are inoperable) |
| Bladder | Surgery, radiotherapy | Fair overall, better if caught early. 50 per cent survival after five years. |
| Prostate | Surgery, radiotherapy | Good, if caught early |

| Testicles | Radiotherapy, surgery | Excellent, if caught early, much less so later |
| Cervix | Surgery, radiotherapy | Good, but the sooner caught the better |
| Womb | Surgery, radiotherapy | Good, 65 per cent survival after five years |
| Ovaries | Surgery | Poor, 25 per cent survival rate after five years |
| Brain | Surgery, radiotherapy | Very poor |
| Sarcomas | Surgery, radiotherapy | Very good |
| Lymphomas | Radiotherapy, chemotherapy | Fair |
| Leukaemia | Chemotherapy, radiotherapy | Good, 70 per cent for acute cases |
| Skin | Surgery, radiotherapy | Good, if treatment not radical (*see note*) |

*Note* In Australia and New Zealand, where melanomas are commonest and surgeons have most experience of treating them, a more conservative approach is taken than the radical surgery common in America. In Queensland, Australia, the five-year survival rate is 81 per cent while in America it is only 37 per cent. In Britain survival rates are 61 per cent.

## Surgery

The surgeon's main role is to cut out tumours that are limited to one site and can be removed without threat to the patient's life, to find out if the cancer has spread to nearby glands, and if so to remove those as well to prevent any further spread.

But surgeons do not just cut out. Part of their job is also to detect and diagnose suspected cancer – first by using their eyes and hands to look at and feel any superficial signs, then, if the growth is inside, to use an endoscope to examine it (*see* 'Endoscopy') and perhaps take a small piece of it for analysis (*see* 'Biopsy').

Once a tumour is known to be malignant, an operation will usually follow pretty quickly, so that no time is lost in removing it. A good surgeon will explain to the patient exactly what is going to be done and why, and what the results are likely to be. The patient will also be asked to sign a consent form beforehand. This signifies that he or she understands what the operation involves, and gives permission for it to be carried out.

In the past cancer surgeons used to remove not only the tumour but also a lot of surrounding tissue. In breast cancer, for example, the whole breast would be removed as well as the glands in the armpit. This was done as a safety measure, and that is still the justification given by those surgeons – mainly in America – who continue to do it.

But the practice began to be heavily criticized when it was found that it often did not increase survival times and sometimes even reduced them – not to speak of the severe psychological problems it caused many women.

Nowadays a good surgeon will only remove as much tissue as is absolutely necessary to avoid disfiguring or mutilating the woman's body. After a lump has been removed from a breast, the breast will sometimes be reconstructed to look as normal as possible.

If the cancer is in a leg bone the better surgeons will now remove the affected bone and replace it with an artificial bone, or *prosthesis*, instead of amputating the leg above the growth as would have happened before.

*Stoma therapy*
Sometimes losing some vital organ in the body is an unavoidable part of even minimum surgery in cancer, but luckily surgeons have become quite skilful at constructing alternative ways of helping the body to continue functioning normally. A good example of this is stoma surgery or therapy.

In cancer of the throat, for instance, the vocal cords usually have to be removed with the growth. Equally, in cancer of the lower bowel much of the gut near the rectum has to be removed, and so the patient can no longer evacuate the bowels normally. Stoma therapy is seen as the solution in both cases.

In the case of the throat operation (*laryngectomy*), the surgeon will make a small permanent hole in the throat, called a *stoma*, into which a tube can be inserted. The patient will be taught how to breathe through this tube, and how to speak in a new way. This is called 'oesophageal speech', and although the voice it produces is rather artificial and strange, the patient can at least speak.

Various mechanical devices have been produced to enable people with laryngectomies to talk and, again, though the voice produced with their aid sounds mechanical and monotonous it is better than no voice at all.

In the case of bowel cancer, if the surgeon cannot join the ends of the intestine together (now done with an instrument resembling a staple gun), he will perform a *colostomy*. He will make a small permanent hole in the wall of the stomach through which he will draw one end of the bowel, to allow it to continue emptying waste matter. A pouch or bag is fitted to the hole to receive the waste, and this can be changed whenever necessary.

It is not easy to adjust to performing a natural function in such an unnatural way, and stoma patients need a lot of help and advice while they are getting used to handling their stomas. Cancer nurses train in stoma therapy so that they can teach patients how to manage their stomas and give them the psychological support they will certainly need in the early stages after operation.

**Case history**

Jane was diagnosed as having breast cancer in her
early 60s after a routine screening test. Jane had been
checking her own breasts for 20 years after having a
benign lump removed and so was shocked to be told
she had breast cancer and would need an operation.

She went into hospital the following week and had
the lump removed. Luckily, the surgeon was able to
leave most of her breast intact. This was followed by
a six-week course of radiotherapy, and a weekend in
hospital having further treatment with radium
implants.

Before the operation Jane was started on the drug
Tamoxifen to block the supply of hormones to her
breasts. Fortunately the cancer had not spread to the
glands in her armpit. Jane returned to the unit for
regular checks and after five years she was pro-
nounced clear.

*Future trends in surgery*
With the aim of making as small a wound as possible,
and of restoring the body to as great a degree of normal-
ity as possible, cancer surgeons are increasingly making
use of the most advanced techniques as a matter of
course. Examples are:

- laser surgery, in which the laser beam passes through
  the tissues without making an incision
- 'keyhole' surgery, in which only a tiny incision is
  made
- microsurgery, using a microscope and extremely small
  instruments to do the most delicate work

In the future, cancer surgeons, like all surgeons, see
themselves becoming experts in robotics, able to perform

operations by remote control. They hope they will also be able to pinpoint tumours, and measure their size and extent, much more precisely with the aid of computerized methods of imaging.

## Radiotherapy

A hundred years ago a Belgian scientist called Roentgen discovered, while he was experimenting with passing a high-voltage current through a vacuum tube, that electromagnetic radiations could penetrate matter. He called these radiations 'X-rays' because he didn't know what they were.

Five years later, in 1900, it was found that these rays could damage human tissue, and could therefore be used, under very careful control, to shrink and even destroy malignant tumours.

(The 'very careful control' is important because clearly if X-rays can damage cancerous tissue – with the aim of killing it – they can also damage healthy tissue. Control of the use of X-rays has been considerably tightened up throughout the Western world in recent years after it was found that many practitioners – not just doctors – were using them too often and at too high a dose.)

Radiotherapy is used to destroy tumours that have been found to be especially sensitive to radiation. It is also used to kill any cancer cells that can remain after surgery and may spread to the glands, as well as to relieve pain and prevent or treat complications when cancer is advanced. This is called 'palliative' treatment. In Britain, more than half of all cancer patients receive radiotherapy.

### How radiotherapy is used in cancer
Radiotherapy can be applied externally, by X-ray machines, or internally, by radioactive implants. External radiation is the most usual method, whether to

shrink the tumour before surgery, to destroy one altogether or to eliminate any cancer cells remaining after surgery. In each case, the dosage required must be calculated very carefully by a physicist in collaboration with a doctor trained in radiotherapy.

Anyone undergoing a course of radiotherapy is likely to come across several sorts of professional with similar names:

- *Radiologists* are doctors specializing in diagnosis.
- *Radiotherapists* are doctors specializing in treatment.
- *Radiographers* are the people who operate the X-ray equipment and give the treatment.

When the dosage has been decided, the course of treatment will be worked out according to the patient's needs. One who can come for treatment every day will have a course of frequent small doses, while one who can only visit the hospital once a week will have higher doses.

Often a machine called a 'simulator' will be used in a sort of rehearsal period before treatment starts, in order to make sure radiation is delivered accurately to the site of the tumour, avoiding healthy tissue. When the head and neck are being treated, Perspex shells are made to cover and protect the patient, holding the part of the body to be irradiated securely in place, allowing the rays to penetrate only to the growth.

Cancers near the surface of the body may be treated by radioactive implants, in the form either of fine needles or of hollow tubes containing radioactive material. These carry radiation directly to the tumour, so the patient has to stay in hospital, isolated from other patients, under strict safety precautions against radioactivity.

*Side-effects*

Radiotherapy does cause side-effects, but these are being reduced by new techniques. The most common side-effect is reddening and irritation of the skin as in sunburn. This builds up towards the end of the course of treatment, but some people react more strongly than others.

Patients also usually feel very tired during treatment, and will need to rest a lot. Sometimes they may feel nauseous, particularly if the stomach and the area round it is being irradiated. Patients should be warned about these side-effects, and given help in coping with them with natural remedies (such as aromatherapy creams and homoeopathy).

If the head and neck are being treated the hair may fall out, though it should start to grow again as soon as the course of treatment ends. If bones containing bone marrow are being irradiated there is a risk that bone marrow (which makes blood) is depressed and this will, in turn, lower resistance to infections. It is therefore important for patients to drink plenty of fluids and eat a really nutritious diet during treatment by radiotherapy to help their bodies heal properly.

*Radiotherapy in the future*

Thanks to computers it is becoming possible for radiotherapists to locate and measure tumours, and target their treatment, much more precisely than before. By the beginning of the next century it is estimated that computerized robots (under doctors' control) may have taken over the whole process of measuring dosages, planning courses of treatment, and delivering the radiation. The theory is that this will make radiotherapy safer and more accurate than it is at present.

## Chemotherapy

The word 'chemotherapy' means treatment by chemicals – in other words, by drugs. The drugs used specifically for cancer are called *cytotoxic* because they poison cells. Their advantage is that they attack cancer cells throughout the entire body (unlike surgery and radiotherapy that destroy cancers only in specific areas). They are therefore very effective in treating cancers which spread throughout the body such as cancers of the blood (eg leukaemia) and the lymphatic system (eg Hodgkin's disease).

### How chemotherapy is used in cancer

Chemotherapy may be used on its own, or in combination with surgery or radiotherapy. It is particularly successful at stopping cancers from spreading from their original site to the glands and other parts of the body, via the circulatory system.

Cytotoxic drugs each have their own individual properties so they may be used on their own, to attack an individual tumour, or in combination with other anticancer drugs in a broad-based assault.

Most anti-cancer drugs can't be taken by mouth like a pill so they are given by injection or by a drip into the vein. A drip is known as an *intravenous infusion* and it is usually done in a hospital or specialist clinic, where nurses give the infusion and doctors can check on the patients' condition and progress.

### Side-effects

Since cytotoxic drugs are all poisonous to rapidly-dividing cancer cells, they affect normal fast-dividing cells such as hair, nails and gut-lining as well, causing side-effects. Patients should be warned of these when the drugs are prescribed for them so that they know they may suffer from nausea and vomiting (if the stomach lining is irritated) or from hair loss (if the hair follicles are damaged).

**Some commonly used anti-cancer drugs**

| Types of cancer | Drug | Common side-effects |
|---|---|---|
| Carcinomas | | |
| Lung | Doxorubicin | Nausea, suppresses bone marrow |
| | Cisplatin | Severe nausea |
| | Methotrexate | Suppresses bone marrow, mucositis, kidney damage |
| Breast | Cyclophosphamide | Cystitis, nausea |
| | Doxorubicin | as above |
| | Methotrexate | as above |
| | Tamoxifen | Hot flushes, dizziness, vaginal bleeding |
| Colon | 5-fluorouracil | Bone marrow suppression |
| Pancreas | 5-fluorouracil | as above |
| Stomach | 5-fluorouracil | as above |
| Testicles | Bleomycin | Lung damage |
| | Cisplatin | as above |
| Ovaries | Cisplatin | as above |
| | Chlorambucil | Bone marrow suppression |
| Prostate | Cyprostat | Liver problems, infertility |
| Bladder | Methotrexate | as above |
| Kidney | Vincristine | Constipation, affects nerves |
| Brain | Vincristine | as above |
| Lymphomas | Bleomycin | as above |
| | Chlorambucil | as above |
| | Cyclophosphamide | as above |
| | Vincristine | as above |
| Leukaemias | Busulfan | Bone marrow suppression |
| | Chlorambucil | as above |
| | Cyclophosphamide | as above |
| Sarcomas | Doxorubicin | as above |
| Childhood cancers | Vincristine | as above |
| | Methotrexate | as above |

The main action of almost all the above drugs is to interfere with cell growth. The exceptions are Cyprostat and Tamoxifen which are used mainly for their hormone-blocking action that affects cell-growth indirectly.

Anti-emetic drugs can help to relieve the nausea and vomiting, and wigs can be worn to conceal baldness during and after treatment (in Britain they are offered free by the state health service). Hair affected by drug therapy normally grows back in time, but it may be of a different colour and texture.

Patients taking anti-cancer drugs may also feel tired and depressed, and have diarrhoea and skin rashes.

Researchers are trying to develop anti-cancer drugs that do not have these unpleasant side-effects, because doctors understand only too well that many patients may decide to stop drug treatment if they can't tolerate the side-effects. But the problem is a big one and solutions hard to find.

## Chemotherapy in the future

Medical scientists researching anti-cancer drugs believe that the advances since the Second World War will accelerate into the next century. The belief is that drugs will be produced that target tumours more accurately and effectively by interfering with the specific biological processes which control growth.

They also expect that response rates to treatment by the new drugs will improve, and side-effects reduced, so that it will be possible to cure many more types of cancer without some of the drastic and unpleasant side-effects currently experienced. The hope is that cancer will no longer be regarded as life threatening, but as a chronic disease that can be kept under control and managed, if not cured.

## Hormone therapy

At the beginning of the century a Scottish doctor called George Beatson found that the flow of milk ewes produced for their lambs was partly controlled by the ovaries. So he removed the ovaries of two women he was treating for very advanced breast cancer to see if this might stop the tumours growing. To his satisfaction the tumour in one woman's breast almost disappeared.

Nowadays an operation to remove the ovaries (*oophorectomy*), which cuts off the supply of hormones to the breasts, is sometimes done to prevent breast cancer spreading or recurring. In men, the testicles may be removed for the same reason, to prevent cancer of the prostate from spreading.

Hormone therapy is used to treat those cancers that are 'hormone-dependent' – that is, they depend on a supply of hormones to help them grow. A laboratory test can tell if a cancer is hormone-dependent. Treatment may be by surgery or by drugs. For example, the drug Tamoxifen blocks the supply of oestrogen to the breasts, and is given to help prevent breast cancer from spreading or from reappearing.

A major trial of the drug is under way in the UK to find out if it will prevent breast cancer developing in healthy women with a family history of breast cancer.

## Summary

Cancer is a life-threatening disease, even if treated. Not only are existing conventional cancer treatments unpleasant and painful, they sometimes fail to cure. Treatment can often seem worse than the disease. The situation is changing, but slowly. Most cancer specialists are committed to 'high-tech' medicine and often fail to see anything of value in gentler, safer therapies such as those offered in natural medicine.

Despite this, cancer units in some hospitals are beginning to make wider use of many of the therapies described in the second half of this book, recognizing that cancer is not just a matter of 'having a tumour' that must be treated but is a disease involving the mental and emotional side of a person as well as the physical.

Often it is the nursing staff rather than the doctors who are showing the most enthusiasm for what is known as the 'holistic' approach. In Britain, for example, the London-based cancer rehabilitation unit of the Royal Marsden cancer hospital is run entirely by nurses trained in a wide range of natural therapies, including massage, relaxation and art. Similar facilities can be found at hospitals in Hammersmith (London), Lancaster and South Cleveland.

But these improvements are still the exception rather than the rule and many people with cancer continue to turn to therapists outside the medical profession for these gentler methods. A survey of patients at the Royal Marsden Hospital in 1990, for example, found that nearly half were seeing a natural therapist to complement the conventional treatment they were receiving.

The difference between the two approaches is perhaps best summed-up by Dr Rosy Daniel, medical director of the Bristol Cancer Help Centre in England: 'Conventional treatments for cancer extend the disease-free period – they don't extend life. Alternative therapies, on the other hand, extend survival time. The difference is clear and important. Conventional medicine puts out the fire – alternative medicine prevents it coming back. The ideal is to get the best of both worlds.'

In the rest of this book we'll outline the gentler methods with the most effective record in helping the 'fire' of cancer returning.

# CHAPTER 6

# The natural therapies and cancer

*Introducing the 'gentle alternatives'*

This book does not say that any natural therapy cures cancer. Such claims have been made for some therapies, and some may be correct. But these claims have not yet been substantiated, at least not in a way acceptable to most conventional scientists. Nevertheless, there are many men and women alive and well today who are convinced that their recovery owes a great deal, if not everything, to their decision to turn to the 'gentle', life-prolonging therapies.

Conventional cancer treatment, as we have seen, relies heavily on three weapons: surgery, radiotherapy and/or chemotherapy. The results in terms of cure or extended survival vary enormously depending on the type of cancer and the stage at which treatment begins. These techniques have their place in cancer treatment but often put the patient under considerable strain and can cause great discomfort.

Natural therapies, such as those described in the following chapters, are based on the idea that cancer can be contained or sometimes even cleared up by giving the body all the help it needs in order to heal itself.

## Why go to a natural therapist?

Surveys have shown that the majority of people with cancer who go to natural therapists do so because they want to try all possible avenues of help or because they want to learn special techniques that will help them cope with their hospital treatment. Very few are abandoning conventional medicine. But a minority may feel that they cannot, or do not want to, face the rigours of conventional treatment for their particular cancer.

People often turn to a natural therapist as a last resort. They have tried the conventional route and it does not seem to have worked. For whatever reason, their needs have not been met and so they no longer want to rely entirely on conventional medical care.

Surveys have shown that more and more people are looking for treatment that is as gentle and non-invasive as possible as well as safe and effective. Rightly or wrongly, they see 'natural medicine' as this sort of approach.

They also do not like the fact that the conventional treatments described in chapter 5 require patients to hand over their care to experts, instead of patients being able to contribute actively to their own recovery. While people appreciate the fact that every effort is being made to cure their physical illness, they feel there isn't time in the conventional scientific medical system to take proper account of the human side of illness.

But the choice in cancer is seldom either/or. Not only is it almost impossible for most cancer patients to avoid conventional treatment in the majority of Western countries, but an increasing number of conventional doctors are aware of the shortcomings of the conventional system and now accept the usefulness of at least some of the natural therapies and make them available to patients.

But how safe are the so-called 'gentle alternatives' and how effective are they really? What is the evidence for their effectiveness? The answers to these questions as far as specific therapies are concerned are in chapters 7 and 8. This chapter deals in general with 'natural' therapy and how it differs from conventional medicine.

## What is natural therapy?

It is a matter of debate (even among therapists themselves) whether all natural therapies share one common idea or principle in the same way that scientific medicine does. Opinions differ, but in general natural therapists do have certain attitudes and principles in common. These can be summarized as:

- The body has a natural ability to heal and regulate itself.
- Each human being is not a random collection of parts but a fully integrated whole. The term 'holistic medicine' is based on this concept and implies treating each patient as a whole being whose intellect and emotions, or spirit, are as important to health as the body.
- Environmental and social conditions have an impact on a person's health.
- Treating the root cause or causes of a problem is more important than tackling the immediate symptoms.
- Each person is unique and cannot be treated in the same way as everyone else.
- It is important to give the patient a sense of their own power and worth, so that they take central responsibility for their own health and are actively involved in the healing process.
- There is a natural healing force in the universe. In the West this is known by the Latin phrase *vis medicatrix naturae* (healing power of nature or 'vital force'), in

China as *qi* or *chi*, in Japan as *ki* and in India as *prana*. Anyone can draw on this healing force: therapists aim to activate it in the patient, or help patients to activate it in themselves.

## The natural therapies and cancer

The natural therapies that have been shown to be helpful for cancer are:

| *Physical therapies* | *Psychological therapies* |
|---|---|
| Acupuncture/acupressure | Art, music, drama therapy |
| Aromatherapy | Counselling |
| Ayurvedic medicine | Healing/faith-healing |
| Homoeopathy | Hypnotherapy |
| Herbalism | Meditation/relaxation |
| Massage | Psychotherapy |
| Naturopathy/hydrotherapy | Visualization (or 'imagery') |
| Nutritional therapy | |
| Reflexology | |
| Yoga and tai chi | |

The most important point for people with cancer is that because cancer is a complex disease with many different causes and symptoms differing from person to person, no one therapy is likely to work on its own – either to see a reduction in the disease or to improve quality of life. Most people who have been helped have found that a combination has worked best.

## Telling your doctor

It is a good idea to tell your doctor that you plan to use natural therapies simply because there may be therapies that are not suitable for particular cancers or which don't mix with particular treatments. For example, it is not advisable to have aromatherapy on a part of the body that is receiving radiotherapy.

Some people are afraid that their doctors will not approve of their wish to complement their treatment with natural therapies. They are afraid that they may show less interest in their case, or even refuse to treat them. This sort of negative resistance is far less likely than it was, thanks to a new generation of enlightened doctors, but sadly it does still exist. If you experience it you should not be afraid to seek another opinion.

Having strong and sympathetic support from a good practitioner is one of the most important weapons in the fight against a disease such as cancer. But don't be put off if your normal doctor asks questions of you.

Any good doctor should be concerned (and most will be) that any therapist you want to consult is properly qualified. That is right and proper and should not be taken as hostility. Nor should it be if he or she wants to refer you to someone else for the same treatment. It is a doctor's role to help guide you to a suitable practitioner and is part of the 'healing partnership' that should exist between a doctor and patient.

Feeling isolated can lead to depression and undermine your recovery programme. Even sufferers who have family and friends around them may find they need more in the way of social support. So a sympathetic and knowledgeable doctor will also be able to tell you if there is a 'support group' in your area. Meeting other people with cancer and sharing your problems with them (as well as listening to theirs) is a good way to understand and overcome difficulties. Some support groups will be familiar with the approaches outlined in this book and sympathetic to them; others will not. Be prepared for either.

Some people fear that meeting fellow-sufferers will add to their worries, but this is rarely the case. You are much more likely to draw strength from each other and enjoy the social activities than suffer from them.

## What to expect from a natural therapist

Just as with your doctor, confidence in and rapport with your therapist is vital. Don't be afraid to ask for credentials or to say 'this therapy or therapist does not feel right for me'. But once you have made your choice 'go for it' wholeheartedly.

Most natural therapists will also encourage you to 'take control' by using such terms as 'taking responsibility for your own health'. Actively participating in your own healing has been shown to be an important factor in the success of most natural therapies and that is why a good practitioner will always encourage you to do this, even if it means just recommending a simple change in lifestyle.

For more on what to expect from a natural therapist and how to find and choose one you can trust *see* chapters 7, 8 and 10.

In some countries there are special centres where diagnosed patients who want to explore the potential of natural therapies can go for a day or longer to find out more about them. In Britain, for example, the Bristol Cancer Help Centre offers residential weeks which include counselling and opportunities to try out certain therapies.

Similarly supportive places are listed in appendix A 'Useful Organizations' at the end of this book. Not the least of the benefits they offer is the chance to meet, in a warm and supportive environment, other people who are in the same boat.

# CHAPTER 7

# Psychological therapies for cancer

*Supporting mind and emotions effectively*

Most leading experts now accept that how you think and feel affects your health. In other words, we know that mental and emotional stresses and strains – or psychological factors, as doctors call them – can make you ill. That means they can trigger cancer, if not even cause it.

How this happens is the object of research in a number of countries, particularly America where the subject has been given the unwieldy name of *psychoneuroimmunology* (PNI), or 'the study of how unhappiness gets into a cell' in the words of British physiologist Dr Clive Wood.

The research focuses on chemicals in the body known as *neuropeptides*. Neuropeptides are vital to the way our brains, glands, intestines and the immune system communicate with each other, and so may also be responsible for communicating feelings and emotions to all parts of the body.

The latest research suggests that neuropeptides may control the growth and spread of tumours and has made the whole field of psychological treatment for cancer come alive.

Though still in its early stages, there are likely to be significant benefits for cancer sufferers as a result of this work in the future. Medicine generally lags about 30 years behind new ideas and discoveries and it may be several more years before all doctors understand and accept the therapies described in this chapter, but few real experts doubt that day is coming.

Psychological therapies of tried and tested benefit in cancer, certainly in alleviating the symptoms and distress it can cause but perhaps also in helping prevent it, are:

- Counselling, including 'attitudinal' and group work
- Psychotherapy and visualization/'imagery'
- Art, music and drama therapies
- Meditation and relaxation
- Healing/faith healing
- Hypnotherapy

Others may emerge in time of equal or greater worth but for the moment these are the therapies where benefit is proven at the hands of skilled and experienced practitioners.

## Facing the diagnosis

It is only recently that attention has been given to one of the most difficult stages in the disease for any cancer sufferer – the diagnosis. Too many sufferers in the past were given a diagnosis, that many saw as a virtual death sentence, and then almost literally turned out into the cold by doctors who did not know to handle the situation and so did nothing about it.

It is now much better understood (though still not enough) that sufferers need most support at the moment of being told they have cancer and for the days immediately after. It is in this situation that psychological support has been shown to be invaluable in helping patients recover their composure and adopt the all-important 'fighting spirit'.

Dr Rosy Daniel, medical director of the Bristol Cancer Help Centre in Britain, for example, has said what she calls 'the kindling of hope' is 'almost always the first step in the recovery process'. It leads, she says, to 'the recovery of fighting spirit, of a sense of control, of emotional and spiritual equilibrium, of self-esteem and personal empowerment'.

This in turn, she says, makes it possible to 'establish a programme of therapy and self-help with clear value both for enhancing life and managing the illness'. Even where there is no dramatic physical improvement, says Dr Daniel, a state of hope makes everything easier – even the contemplation of death itself.

Realizing that often someone will not take in what is said after hearing the dread word 'cancer' some doctors now tape the whole conversation and give a copy of the tape to the patient to take away and play at home.

In most Western countries good cancer centres have trained specialists, usually nurses or counsellors, available to give help and advice to cancer patients.

There are national telephone 'helplines' in many countries also (*see* appendix A). Helpline organizations may offer the opportunity for face-to-face counselling by appointment at their own premises or give out the names of accredited counsellors practising in the enquirer's home district.

## Counselling

Counselling is the process of talking things over with a skilled and understanding listener called a counsellor to re-evaluate your lifestyle and values. In cancer this can ease any sense of isolation you may be feeling and reveal unexpected sources of strength and hope.

Counselling offers two vital things: time for yourself and someone who really listens to what you say. This is what makes it work. One way in which counselling (and psychotherapy, *see* page 88) can be helpful to newly diagnosed cancer patients, for example, is that it can help them to identify and resolve any feelings that they may be harbouring of guilt, self-blame or resentment towards others.

Cancer brings all sorts of emotions to the surface such as fear, anger, sadness and guilt. These can be distressing to yourself and those nearest to you. Talking about what is happening can help you to begin to untangle the confusions and uncertainties that cancer brings.

The goal is to help each person find their own unique way of coping creatively so that they can emerge happier and stronger, often with a clearer sense of purpose and commitment to life than before their illness.

A good counsellor will not tell you what to do but may offer suggestions to point you towards new ways of coping and perhaps help you to find new ways of saying things that you have found hard to say to those close to you. The counsellor will aim to 'be there' with you and be a 'mirror' in which you can see yourself more clearly.

Different counsellors have different styles and approaches to their work and so it is important to find one you feel at ease with and relaxed. Most counsellors want to be sure that the help they can offer is appropriate for the individual concerned so it is quite usual to have one or two trial sessions before committing to more. If it doesn't seem to be working well with that particular counsellor a good professional should always be happy to refer to another who might be better suited to your needs.

## Pioneers of psychological treatments for cancer

There is nothing new about the idea that mind and emotions can cause cancer. Centuries ago Hippocrates, the Greek 'father of medicine', said that 'melancholic' women were more likely to get breast cancer than others.

Wise physicians down the centuries remained aware of the mind-body connection but the idea became overshadowed in the 18th and 19th centuries as scientists concentrated on how the body worked. It was not until the late 20th century that doctors as a whole began to rediscover the link. Among the first was American psychologist Dr Lawrence LeShan who associated cancer with traumatic events such as bereavement and divorce in the 1950s. By 1982 it was believed that emotional loss in childhood could predispose an adult to cancer. A study of students at an American university, for example, revealed that those who developed cancer in later life had described their parents as 'cold and distant', and had found it difficult to express their feelings to them.

During the 1980s also, defining the 'cancer personality' became fashionable. People with this personality were those who felt insecure, inadequate or guilty, repressed normal emotions of love or aggression, and reacted to life's problems and tragedies with silent stoicism or self-blame.

The theory, that this repression of feeling eventually finds an outlet by allowing malignant tumours to grow, found support in 1987 when American psychiatrist David Spiegel showed that women with breast cancer who attended a support group and learnt a relaxation technique lived twice as long as another group who did not do so.

Other American pioneers of the 1980s were Dr Norman Cousins, Dr Gerry Jampolsky, Dr Deepak Chopra and Dr Bernie Siegel – all of whom were concerned with the power of 'negative' thinking to make disease more likely or worse and of 'positive' thinking to prevent, halt and even cure it. Researchers in other countries, notably Britain and Australia, followed suit.

In Australia, Melbourne psychiatrist Dr Ainslie Meares claimed that deep relaxation could cure cancer, while in Britain, psychiatrist Dr Steven Greer followed the progress of 62 women cancer patients for 15 years in a project known as the Courtauld Follow-up Study, and found that those with 'fighting spirit' survived longer than those who felt helpless and 'gave in'.

In another study by Dr Greer, newly diagnosed cancer patients who went on a specially designed programme of short-term psychological therapy showed greater improvement than those who did not.

More recently, American PNI expert Dr Candace Pert, of Georgetown University School of Medicine, has shown that emotional states not only affect immune function but the growth of cancer cells.

This view seems to have been confirmed in 1995 in a joint UK–Taiwanese study at King's College Hospital, London, that found a strong link between severe mental and emotional distress and the development of breast cancer. The study of the psychological aspects of cancer now has its own name in conventional medicine – 'psycho-oncology'.

## Psychotherapy

Psychotherapy is nothing to do with psychiatry, a conventional medical discipline that uses drugs (and, rarely, surgery) to treat mental and emotional problems. Psychotherapists use a variety of techniques, but the emphasis is on discussion rather than drugs or surgery.

Psychotherapy has much in common with counselling and in broad terms psychotherapy is a more involved form of counselling. Counsellors deal with problems in the here and now whereas psychotherapists are more concerned with deep-seated emotional hurts. This may mean delving into past experiences to discover and discuss any unconscious conflicts.

In cancer, the most effective psychotherapies are those that explore and attempt to resolve painful or conflicting thoughts and emotions. The aim is to build up a sense of psychological well-being and so reinforce the patient's physical defences.

The following are sometimes suggested in the treatment of cancer:

- art therapies
- laughter therapy
- relaxation therapy
- visualization therapy
- Transpersonal psychology

### Art therapies

This is a general term for therapies that use various artistic techniques to let people express their innermost feelings without having to put them into words as they do for a counsellor. Art therapies can include painting, music, drama, movement, dance – and in fact any method that allows the full expression of thoughts and emotions. They are available on an individual or group basis.

### Laughter therapy

Work with cancer patients, particularly in Sweden, has shown that making the most of opportunities to laugh is one of the most powerful ways of building up psychological well-being. American journalist Norman Cousins twice fought so successfully against critical illness by making himself watch Laurel and Hardy films he wrote a book about it – and then qualified as a doctor to allow him to teach his ideas to others.

Such a near-miracle is beyond the powers of most people with cancer, though, and help in this area is almost always best sought from a therapist working with a group.

### Relaxation therapy

Relaxation is another powerful way to overcome unhealthy stresses and strains and is easily learnt as self-help (*see* chapter 4). Most experts see it as the process of 'going within'. In other words, it's about using a variety of ways to gain access to a deeper level of consciousness. At this level the mind becomes quiet in a way that even sleep doesn't bring.

Research over the years, particularly in America by Dr Herbert Benson and more recently by doctors working with meditation at the Maharishi International University, has shown that deep relaxation can have a profound effect on the body, significantly lowering blood pressure, among other processes.

Specialists say that whatever method works best for you is the best method to use, but a good psychotherapist should be able to advise on a wide range of relaxation techniques. Among those most likely to be recommended are exercise, massage, yoga and meditation.

#### Meditation

Meditation is the process of allowing the mind to become quiet and focused and is well established as accelerating the healing process in a wide range of conditions. It is particularly beneficial when used alongside other natural therapies.

You can meditate on your own or in a group. Teaching is so widely available these days that it is quite likely your local library or information centre will include such groups in its list of local societies. A Westernised version of the Oriental types familiar to most people is *autogenic training*.

Autogenic – the word means 'generated from within' – training is a technique which aims to bring a profound sense of relaxation and relief from the negative effects of stress. It is said to work by bringing the two sides of the brain into balance and to support the natural healing mechanisms.

The therapy involves a series of mental and physical exercises and can be particularly helpful for people who have difficulty with traditional meditative techniques. It is normally learnt in groups at a hospital or private centre. A typical course would involve about eight once-a-week sessions, after which you should be able to do it as self-help wherever you happen to be as no special equipment is necessary.

## Visualization therapy

Another good method of building up psychological well-being, visualization – or 'imagery' as it is sometimes called – is a therapy in which patients are taught to picture in their 'mind's eye' positive health-promoting images. This is believed to help along natural healing processes and reinforce positive behaviour.

The technique is used to help patients suffering from a wide range of conditions, including cancer. It, too, can be practised quite easily as a form of self-help (*see* chapter 4) but many people find it better to start off with someone skilled in teaching 'creative visualization' or offering 'guided imagery'.

Some therapists use paintings by famous artists as an aid to visualization. After looking at a painting for a few minutes, the patient is asked to recall it with their eyes shut. After a while, people usually find they are able to 'see' more and more of the details and this practice helps them to visualize a real-life situation more easily.

In cancer care, for example, the patient may visualize the tumour being attacked and destroyed, or melting away and disappearing. The technique can be particularly useful when a patient is undergoing radiotherapy or chemotherapy. Fewer side-effects have been noted when it is used.

## Healing

Healing, also known as 'faith healing' or 'spiritual healing', is not strictly-speaking a psychological therapy so much as a psychic one. Its practitioners (*see* figure 5) believe they are healing someone by transferring or 'channelling' some sort of unknown power or energy from or through themselves to the person being healed.

But to claim to be able to heal by the use of such powers is illegal in some countries, particularly in parts of America and Germany, and so it is instead seen as a legitimate form of 'mind–body' therapy. In America, for example, it is better known as 'Therapeutic Touch' (or 'TT').

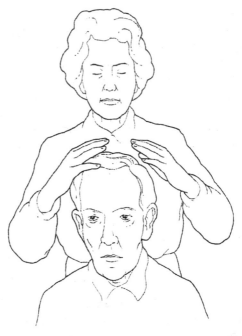

**Fig. 5　A healer at work**

Whether there is an external force at work or not, there is substantial evidence that healing does have an effect, and even if this is only because the person being treated has faith that they are being healed it is not to be overlooked. In cancer, anything that works is worth encouraging and there is substantial evidence that healing causes a reduction in fear levels.

People who claim to be able to heal far outnumber all other natural therapists put together so finding a healer is not hard these days. Finding a good one is harder and the rule is to act on recommendation. More guidance on how to find and choose a good therapist is in chapter 10.

## Hypnotherapy

Hypnotherapy or hypnosis is a state of relaxation and concentration which a person enters so that the deeper parts of the mind can become more accessible. In cancer care it is used for pain relief and to promote relaxation before treatments or investigative procedures. There is also considerable evidence that hypnotherapy can reduce nausea after chemotherapy and can make patients better able to deal with the physical and emotional impact of cancer.

Care is needed when choosing a therapist outside a supervised setting such as a hospital or clinic, but research has shown that people under hypnosis do not say or do anything against their will – in spite of the impression given by stage performers.

## Summary

Psychological therapies for cancer usually work best in combination with therapies that concentrate on treating the physical aspects (discussed in the next chapter).

# CHAPTER 8

# Physical therapies for cancer

*Supporting the body effectively*

Natural physical therapies concentrate on supporting the person's immune system and alleviating the side-effects of disease and any conventional treatments being undergone.

However, it is important to understand that none of the natural therapies *on its own* can *cure* cancer. The main role of these therapies is in alleviation and support, and in this they can be highly effective. Therapies that help the patient to relax and deal with stress are particularly useful.

The main physical therapies useful in cancer care are:

- Acupuncture and acupressure
- Aromatherapy
- Ayurveda
- Homoeopathy
- Herbalism
- Massage
- Naturopathy/Hydrotherapy
- Nutritional therapy
- Reflexology
- Yoga and t'ai chi

## Acupuncture

Acupuncture is an ancient Chinese therapy used to treat a wide variety of conditions, but in cancer care it is used to relieve nausea and pain, especially when the tumour presses on a nerve.

Acupuncture is routinely used in Chinese hospitals as an anaesthetic, often combined with Chinese herbs or Western drugs. These days it is commonly used in the West in conventional pain clinics as well as by individual doctors and practitioners trained in Oriental medicine.

According to Chinese philosophy acupuncture works by releasing the 'life force', or *chi* energy, which controls the main organs and systems of the body. The energy moves from one organ to another along 14 pathways or 'meridians' (*see* figure 6). Fine needles made of stainless steel or gold are inserted into one or more of the 400 or so acupuncture points it is believed lie along these meridians and agitated to encourage the release or flow of energy.

Research has shown that the needles, when inserted into the points and manipulated, release chemicals called *endorphins* into the bloodstream. Endorphins are natural painkillers. Another theory is that the needle stimulation blocks nerve pathways that carry pain signals to the brain.

A variation of acupuncture with needles is *moxibustion*. Moxibustion is the application of heat from a slow-burning herb known as *moxa*, held near or above the acupuncture point or the diseased part of the body. The heat can be applied by a smouldering stick or cone of the herb or attached to the needle itself so that the heat transfers to the body down the needle. Another widespread variation is *acupressure*. In acupressure (which may be even older than acupuncture) the release of energy is done by pressing the points with the fingertips. A Japanese version well known in the West is *shiatsu* (shiatsu means 'finger pressure' in Japanese).

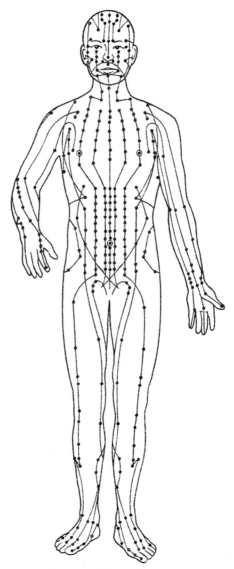

**Fig. 6 The acupuncture meridians**

## Aromatherapy

Aromatherapy or 'smell therapy' is best known in cancer care for its effectiveness as a relaxant when the sweet-smelling plant oils it is based on are combined with massage.

The medicinal properties of plant essences (or 'essential oils') have been known for thousands of years but it was not until earlier this century that the art was revived by a French chemist, René-Maurice Gattefosse, who discovered the healing power of lavender oil after plunging his badly burned hand into it. The burn healed quickly, without a scar.

Gattefosse successfully treated soldiers wounded in the First World War with lavender and other healing oils and soon the idea spread from France to Britain and thence to the rest of the world.

Essential oils can be applied in a number of ways and though their use in massage is the best known they can also be inhaled and used in baths or compresses. Specialists even use certain oils internally. The oils themselves have no known curative powers for cancer, however.

*Caution* In cancer massage should not be given over the site of a tumour or to the surrounding tissue in case it spreads the cancer. Never drink essential oils without expert guidance and don't use them undiluted. It is wise to consult a qualified *clinical* aromatherapist in the first place (beauty therapists who do massage don't have the right skills) but you can learn how to use the wide variety of oils available at home.

## Ayurvedic medicine

Ayurveda is not one therapy but a whole system of medicine which originated in India and has now also become popular in the West. Yoga, for example, is an ayurvedic technique. The name ayurveda is derived from two Sanskrit words and means 'the science or knowledge of life'.

Great emphasis is placed on prevention of disease in ayurveda, but when illness occurs practitioners use a wide variety of remedies and techniques, especially plant-based drugs and mineral supplements. As in all natural, and especially Oriental, therapies, its practitioners find out a great deal about the patient before prescribing treatment.

In cancer care, the ayurvedic approach can be used supportively to ease stress and tension. The system has won the respect of many Western doctors and a number of them practise ayurvedic medicine alongside their conventional medicine.

## Homoeopathy

This is another of those therapies with allegedly ancient roots that has been rediscovered. This time the discovery was made by an 18th-century German physician, Samuel Hahnemann, who found taking quinine (an anti-malaria drug) when he was well gave him the symptoms of malaria. This led him to do research from which he developed the theory of 'like cures like' that is the basis of homoeopathy to this day.

According to homoeopathy, a substance that *causes* certain symptoms in a healthy person will *cure* the same or similar symptoms in a person sick with symptoms of that disease.

Homoeopathic remedies are derived from plant, mineral or animal sources and are carefully matched to the patient. They are 'potentized' by being diluted over and over again until only tiny amounts of the original substance remain and shaken vigorously – or 'succussed' – at every dilution.

This concept of 'the weaker the stronger' is so foreign to conventional scientific thinking that the use of homoeopathy in cancer care is extremely controversial. Because no one is agreed yet how homoeopathy actually works (one theory is that the very dilute substances used in homeopathy somehow leave 'footprints' in water) some doctors think any benefits are purely psychosomatic or 'placebo'. That is, you feel better because you believe you are better and for no other reason.

In some American states opposition is so strong homoeopathy is actually banned as being somehow connected with witchcraft. By contrast, it is widely practised by doctors in several European countries, notably France and Germany, and increasingly widely available throughout the world.

In Britain, where it is recognized by the state health service, there are five homoeopathic hospitals and around a thousand doctors trained in it. The therapy has long been popular with the British royal family. Queen Elizabeth, for example, has a personal homoeopathic physician and always takes homoeopathic remedies with her when travelling.

The Royal London Homoeopathic Hospital has developed a 'package of care' for people with cancer referred by their family doctor. The treatment combines massage, relaxation and homoeopathic medicines prescribed by specialists, who see the programme as supporting patients' conventional treatment.

## Massage

Hippocrates wrote 'the way to health is to have a scented bath and an oiled massage each day' and massage can become a vital ingredient at a deep level in a person's process of becoming and staying healthy.

A trial in 1995 by nurses at London's Royal Marsden

Hospital showed that pain and anxiety were significantly reduced in cancer patients receiving massage against those who did not. Massage, adapted for cancer patients, can also provide an opportunity to 'let go' emotionally and can help to restore a healthy sleep pattern.

Although massage is a perfectly safe as well as effective therapy (and is now in regular use in leading cancer centres, including Professor Karol Sikora's famous unit in Hammersmith, London) care must be taken not to massage the actual site of a tumour or any parts of the body made tender by cancer or its treatment.

## Medical herbalism

Medical herbalism – the use of plants or plant materials to treat disease and to promote health – is probably the oldest form of medicine. It can be traced back to early Egyptian times (4000 BC) and was probably widespread thousands of years before that. Until recently it was the dominant therapy in every society on earth.

It is only this century that the majority of medicines used by doctors have become synthetic chemicals rather than herbs. Though many modern drugs are also plant based, drugs are isolated extracts of parts of plants. Herbalists use whole plants because they believe whole plants have a natural balance that increases their healing powers, as well as making them easier for the body to use, and counteracts side-effects.

Among herbs that have been used in cancer care are silymarin, echinacea and two Brazilian herbs: suma and pau d'arco. Iscador, an extract of mistletoe, is thought to be toxic to cancer cells and to increase immune-system function.

American healer Harry Hoxsey made up herbal recipes for which anti-cancer claims have been made but there is only anecdotal evidence for these claims and no proof. Equally, claims have been made that herbs used in Chinese medicine relieve the side-effects of conventional cancer treatments but so far there have been no independent tests of this and most doctors have their doubts.

Sceptics, however, say that herbal remedies for cancer are unlikely to become established because any that do offer significant benefits will immediately be turned by the pharmaceutical industry into a patented drug.

*Caution* Herbs, like all medicines, can cause problems if used wrongly. There is a risk that some herbs may interact dangerously with cancer drugs so be sure to consult a qualified herbalist before trying any (*see* chapter 10 for how to find one you can rely on).

## Naturopathy

This, like ayurveda, is not a single therapy but another general approach to the treatment of ill-health based on the principle that the body has a natural inbuilt ability to heal itself. Naturopathy (also known as 'nature cure' and 'natural hygiene') has much in common with traditional Indian and Chinese medicine.

Naturopaths believe that disease arises when the body's natural self-regulating processes are 'below par' or have been compromised in some way and so concentrate on a variety of techniques to restore the natural balance and so return the body to health.

Stress, poor diet, pollution and lack of exercise have all long been seen by naturopaths as upsetting the natural balance or *homeostasis* and many naturopathic techniques emphasize cleansing the body of the waste products and toxins they believe are caused by unhealthy lifestyle and living conditions.

A practitioner will aim to get a complete picture of the patient by detailed history-taking and will usually also give a medical examination similar to that given by a conventional doctor. Among treatments likely to be recommended in cancer are special diets, brief fasting, herbal remedies and nutritional supplements.

Naturopaths usually train at specialist colleges in a range of skills that include acupuncture, herbalism, hydrotherapy (using water), homoeopathy and nutritional therapy.

Except in Britain, naturopathy is becoming the standard training for those interested in practising natural medicine in its widest sense. Countries such as the United States, Canada, Australia, Germany, Israel, New Zealand and South Africa run full three- to four-year courses leading to a recognized degree of doctor of naturopathy.

In spite of this training, naturopaths are not medical doctors and so the same cautions apply as elsewhere in this chapter when consulting a naturopath about cancer treatment.

## Nutritional therapy

Research evidence to show that diet and food supplements have a vital role in both the prevention of cancer and as an aid to recovery is now overwhelming – so much so that in September 1995 the European Commission's Europe Against Cancer programme was officially forecasting that a cancer prevention diet would be available by 1998.

In another recent major development the Bristol Cancer Help Centre in Britain announced a computerized database with details of over 5,000 studies published in mainstream scientific journals between 1983 and 1994 showing the links between diet and cancer. Although a number of natural therapies are advocated by the centre, good nutrition is at the heart of its philosophy, according to medical director Dr Rosy Daniel.

The claims for nutritional therapy in cancer are that it improves nutritional status and energy levels, reduces side-effects of chemotherapy and radiotherapy, helps to control some cancer symptoms and assists the body's immune and repair processes.

---

**Some studies showing links between diet and cancer**

- A 19-year study of 3,000 men showed that men with low levels of beta-carotene (a precursor of vitamin A) had a seven- to eightfold greater risk of lung cancer than those with high levels.
- A 1992 Spanish study of breast cancer and diet linked a lower death rate from cancer with a decrease in blood fats and increased intake of fibre, cereals and vitamin C.
- Finnish research in 1991 on 36,000 men showed that those with low levels of vitamin E had a one and a half times greater risk of cancer than those with higher levels.
- An American study in 1992 of 11,000 men showed that high vitamin C intake links strongly with low cancer death rates.

All studies taken from the Bristol Cancer Help Centre database, England.

---

Evidence is also growing for the role of a wholefood diet and vitamins and minerals to support conventional treatment by radiotherapy, chemotherapy and surgery. Researchers have found speedier recovery from operations, with fewer post-operative complications and infections.

Although what is included and excluded varies, the dietary programmes recommended by natural therapists follow more or less the diet now approved by most conventional doctors and described in chapter 4.

Some specialists in cancer therapy, however, go further and prescribe very specific diets they believe (and indeed claim) can actively cure cancer. Among those widely promoted in the past, especially in America, have been the Hoxsey diet, the Block diet, the Livingston-Wheeler diet, the Gerson diet and the macrobiotics diet, but only the last two have, so far, produced any convincing evidence for their claims.

### Gerson therapy

The Gerson diet or 'Gerson therapy' is perhaps the best known of the strict dietary regimes for cancer. Devised by the late Max Gerson (a German doctor who migrated to America) to help cope with his own migraine, the therapy is now controlled by the Gerson Institute with headquarters in California.

The regime, which includes counselling as an integral part of the therapy, is demanding and time consuming and despite criticism from the National Cancer Institute and the American Cancer Society, it continues to have a wide following and to claim results. The individual nature of many of the results, though, makes it difficult to test the claims scientifically and a much-publicized 15-year survey of its success with melanoma, published in September 1995, has yet to be supported. Other independent studies on the Gerson therapy have been inconclusive.

One problem facing would-be researchers is the important part played in such regimes by the individual patient's commitment. The standard randomized clinical trial is not relevant in this situation.

### Macrobiotics

This is a slightly less rigid diet based on an ancient Oriental approach of 'food balancing' recently popularized in the West by Michio Kushi, a Japanese political scientist now based in America. It is widely followed by many people who are healthy as well as those who are ill.

To follow the diet properly requires an understanding of the degree to which foods are *yin* or *yang* (*see box*). Sweet foods and alcohol, for example, are believed to be extremely yin, while meat, eggs, cheese and dairy produce are very yang. In between come the foods from which the macrobiotic diet is selected: grains, vegetables, fruit, sea vegetables and soya products.

Little research seems to have been done on the anti-cancer effects of the macrobiotic diet but it does feature many foods thought to be beneficial in the prevention and alleviation of cancer. Fore more details, refer to the books by Michio Kushi such as *The Book of Macrobiotics*, (Japan Publications, 1987).

---

**Yin and yang**

These are the two opposing but complementary forces which the ancient Chinese believed governed all aspects of life, including medicine. Yin was seen as more passive, yang as the more positive, thrusting force. The first book classifying medical symptoms and treatments according to the principle of yin–yang balance was compiled by Chang Chung-ching around AD 200. Disease is said to result when a person's yin and yang are not in balance, so treatment seeks to build up whichever of the two forces is weaker. Diet is only one of many natural therapies that may be employed to achieve this.

---

### Megavitamin supplementation

Many natural therapists prescribe antioxidant nutrients such as vitamins A, C and E, the mineral selenium and the so-called 'essential fatty acids', among others, in the fight against cancer (*see* page 106).

Supplementation for cancer using very high doses is known as 'super-nutritional therapy' or 'megavitamin therapy'. Positive research results have been reported from studies into megavitamin therapy, particularly the use of vitamin C, in Scotland, the United States and Canada, but so far the therapy has only been assessed for its usefulness alongside conventional cancer treatments.

---

**Suggested supplement levels for people with cancer**

| Nutrient | For active cancer | For prevention/ maintenance |
| --- | --- | --- |
| Vitamin A or | 10,000iu | 7,500iu |
| beta-carotene (preferable) | 25,000iu | 10,000iu |
| Vitamin B complex | 50mg | 50mg |
| Vitamin C | 6–10g | 1–3g |
| Vitamin E | 200–400iu | 100iu |
| Zinc (elemental) | 15–25mg | 15mg |
| Selenium | 200mcg | 100mcg |
| Chromium GTF | 100mcg | 50mcg |
| Magnesium | 100–200mg | 100–200mg |

From 'Nutritional and Lifestyle Guidelines for People with Cancer', *Journal of Nutritional Medicine*, 1994 (4, 199–214). *Note* There is a considerable difference between the doses recommended to prevent cancer and those to fight it. The doses listed above and in chapter 4 for self-help are for prevention only. To fight cancer doses need to be many times higher and self-prescription is not recommended as there is a real danger of overdoing the amounts in some cases. Supplementation for cancer should really only be carried out under the supervision of an experienced practitioner.

---

### Reflexology

This is another of the supportive therapies which, in cancer care, aims to improve the patient's well-being and stimulate the immune system. Modern reflexology is believed to be based on ancient healing practices with possible links to Chinese medicine.

## Ian Gawler's story

Australian vet Ian Gawler claims to have cured himself of advanced bone cancer – resulting in him losing a leg in 1975 and being given just two weeks to live at one stage – with a mixture of detoxification, correcting various vitamin and mineral imbalances in his body, and a diet of fresh, pure food coupled with intense meditation, a positive attitude and loving support.

Since his progressive recovery in the 1980s he has become a leading exponent of the holistic approach to cancer treatment. He has set up the Gawler Foundation in Melbourne, offering a nutritional programme combined with psychological therapies such as meditation, and runs the Yarra Valley Living Centre with his wife Grace, a veterinary nurse and qualified herbalist.

Pressure is put on the feet, usually with the thumbs, to stimulate nerve endings which it is believed are linked to all the body organs (*see* figure 7). Some reflexologists work on the hands, arms and legs as well. 'Energy lines' similar to the meridians in Chinese medicine run from the feet, up to the head and down to the hands. Any discomfort or pain on the point being pressed is said to indicate a problem in the corresponding area of the body. This may be uncomfortable at first but the pain usually eases and a response is felt in the affected organ.

There are a few variants, such as Reflex Zone Therapy, Morrell Reflexology and Vacuflex (a hi-tech version using a vacuum pump and suction pads), but all methods are widely acknowledged to be perfectly safe and to produce usually a feeling of intense relaxation.

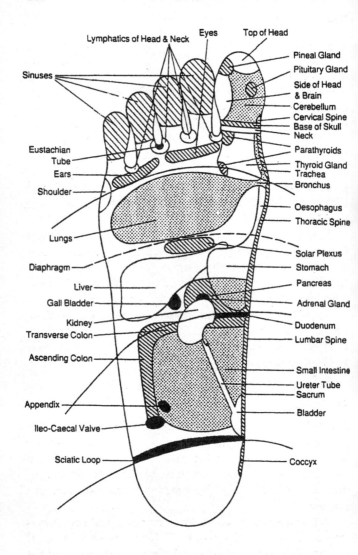

**Fig. 7 Reflex zones on the right foot**

## Yoga

Yoga is an ancient spiritual discipline with profound therapeutic benefits. Originating in India, where it forms a major part of ayurveda (*see* page 97), it combines movement and posture with correct breathing. Breath control is important in yoga because the philosophy behind it regards breath as containing *prana* or life force.

Yoga is now so popular and widespread throughout the Western world it should not be difficult to find a class by a qualified teacher. In a 1983 survey in Britain of people practising yoga conducted by the Yoga Biomedical Trust 90 per cent of those with cancer said they had benefited.

There are similarities between yoga and *qi gong*, a Chinese system of exercises currently becoming popular in the West. The graceful art of t'ai chi – often called 'meditation in motion' and a common sight in Chinese cities early in the morning – is a form of qi gong.

Yoga, t'ai chi and chi kung all encourage relaxation and counter stress. But it is important to find teachers who are well qualified and who conduct a quiet and well-ordered class for maximum benefit.

## Summary

A combination of natural therapies that treat both the physical and psychological aspects of the disease are likely to play an increasing part in cancer care and self-help as evidence continues to mount that all those covered in this book can be as effective as they are safe and gentle.

But no treatment works for everybody and sometimes improvement is not possible. Taking a positive look at the situation when cure is unlikely is the purpose of the next chapter.

# CHAPTER 9

# When treatment fails to cure

*Help and care for the dying*

There comes a time in some cases of cancer when it is clear that medically speaking the disease is incurable – although pioneers in cancer care stress that just because a doctor thinks so or says so does not mean it is so. In cancer nothing is certain and keeping a positive 'fighting' spirit is often crucial.

When doctors think that death is inevitable they are faced with the dilemma of whether or not to tell the patient. It is a dilemma that has been debated by professional carers for many years. Some believe it is kinder not to tell patients they are dying, but to tell the relatives instead. Others – probably the majority now – believe the patient should be told the truth.

How this should be done is equally open to debate at the moment but the majority favour telling patients in very easy and gentle stages, according to how much they can face up to at one time. Experience has shown that after patients have gone through the natural stages of shock, disbelief, anger, grief and despair, they are able to share their feelings with their relatives or close friends, face the future together, and make practical plans to put their affairs in order – emotionally as well as practically.

## Case history

Lewis Chapman, 78, had been treated for prostate cancer in hospital, and had been warned it might return as bone cancer, although he was given the choice of an *orchidectomy* (removal of the testicles) as a preventive measure, which he accepted.

He did not tell his wife that he had had cancer or that it might return, for fear of worrying her. He appeared to make a good recovery and there was no sign of further trouble. But then he began getting severe pain in his hipjoints and lower back. He went back to hospital for tests, and was told he had osteoarthritis of the spine. He was given drugs to kill the pain and reduce the inflammation in his joints.

His condition did not improve and, becoming very worried the cancer might have returned, he asked his neighbour, who worked in medicine, whether this might be so. She knew it was likely but could not say so. Instead she spoke to the couple's daughter, suggesting she find out the truth from their family doctor.

The doctor visited Mr Chapman, asking the family to be present too, and explained to them that the cancer had returned in his bones and could not be cured. He also told them that he would admit Mr Chapman to the local hospice if they couldn't manage to nurse him at home.

Although they all felt great shock and sadness, they were relieved to know the truth and to be able to discuss it frankly. Mr Chapman stayed at home as long as possible, and died a peaceful death a few weeks later in the hospice, with his wife and family around him.

The story of Mr Chapman is, sadly, a common one where cancer is concerned. Death does happen. But of course death is not, as some people would like it to be, an optional extra: it happens to us all. It is a part of life and something everyone has to face sooner or later. Most people naturally find it difficult to accept the idea of dying, but many of those who are dying of cancer say it is not death they fear so much as the process of dying, especially the thought of a prolonged and painful struggle.

In professional cancer care, doctors and nurses live with the reality of death all the time. As a result they have given a great deal of thought to controlling and managing the symptoms that can occur in the advanced stages of cancer so as to keep people as comfortable as possible and their quality of life as good as possible until the end.

## Symptom control

The symptoms that occur most commonly in the late stages of cancer are pain, breathlessness, nausea and loss of appetite, incontinence (or constipation and retention of urine), and weakness. There can be others, according to the type of cancer, but these are the main ones.

### Pain

A frequent cause of cancer pain is that the growth is pressing on a nerve or an organ, but the pain may be caused by an infection or by another condition such as arthritis or heart disease. The types of pain vary from a dull ache to a sharp shooting pain, and may need to be treated differently.

Pain is usually controlled by drugs. Doctors believe that chronic pain should never be allowed to surface, so big enough doses of painkilling drugs are given at regular intervals to keep the pain under control at all times. Though powerful drugs like morphine are addictive or habit forming this is not seen as mattering at this stage of the disease.

Radiotherapy is sometimes given to relieve bone pain, and when the pain is local, the nerve may be blocked by injecting an anaesthetic at the site.

Many of the natural therapies described in the last chapter, such as acupuncture and acupressure, can also be very effective in relieving pain and giving patients comfort at this stage of their lives. Others useful for pain relief include art therapy, imagery, relaxation, massage, aromatherapy and reflexology.

### Nausea and vomiting

These distressing symptoms can affect people suffering from all types of cancer, not just of the stomach and intestines. They may be the result of treatment, or of psychological distress.

Whatever the cause, nausea and vomiting can be controlled by 'antiemetic' drugs – drugs that prevent vomiting. If the patient can't swallow a pill the drugs are given by injection or by suppositories (a gel pessary inserted into the rectum).

Alternatives are acupuncture and hypnosis. Both have been shown by research to be effective at controlling nausea and vomiting.

### Breathlessness

There can be several different causes of breathlessness and conventional treatment is usually with drugs, depending on the cause. For example:

- Drugs that expand a narrowed airway (*bronchodilators*) are used if there is spasm in the lungs.
- Antibiotics are used to treat an infection.

- Corticosteroids may be used for obstruction of the lungs.
- Diuretics or digoxin are for heart failure.

Patients are usually nursed sitting up, as they can breathe more easily in an upright position, and are given comfort and reassurance to allay their natural anxiety.

Of the natural therapies, relaxation and breath control are the most helpful with breathlessness.

## *Constipation*

This is a very common symptom, and can be caused by drugs. Because it is very important that constipation is properly dealt with in cancer care, it is treated by preparations that either soften the stools or create bulk, making it easier to pass them out of the bowel, or by drugs that draw water into the intestines, or stimulate what is called *peristaltic movement* – the involuntary contractions of the bowel that expel the stools.

Suppositories may also be used to get rid of any hard *faeces* (stools) that have collected and are blocking the bowel. But high fibre foods and herbal preparations such as psyllium husks can be just as good.

Aromatherapy massage with marjoram or rose in a base oil can help to relieve constipation when applied to the lower back and reflexology is also said to help.

## *Incontinence and urine retention*

The bladder sometimes stops working normally in the late stages of cancer. This is usually because it is linked to a part of the body affected by the cancer, but it can also be a side-effect of drugs. Retention of urine is usually treated by inserting a tube to draw off the urine, and there is a large range of pads, pants and other equipment to cope with incontinence. For carers it is as well to know that incontinent patients should be able to reach a toilet easily, so that they don't suffer the humiliation of soiling themselves.

## Weakness and weight loss

This is the most common symptom of all, and can be due to drugs, loss of sleep, loss of appetite, nausea and vomiting, and pain. Attempting to maintain weight is crucial in cancer, and almost all the natural therapies mentioned in this book score well here. Nurses and volunteers trained in care of the dying may be trained in one or more of them nowadays. A 1994 survey showed that 90 per cent of hospices and palliative care units in Britain now offer some kind of touch therapy such as massage, aromatherapy or reflexology.

## The place to die

If death is unexpected it can happen anywhere and at any time. But if it is expected choices can be made.

Hospitals can be intimidating places and many people would prefer to die at home, in their own familiar surroundings, near to those whom they love and who love them. Often community-based care workers can help make this possible for those too in awe of doctors and their ways.

These days there is now a third choice – the hospice. A hospice is a type of nursing home that specializes in caring for the dying and in making what remains of their lives as easy and comfortable as possible. Originally founded in Britain, the hospice movement has now spread round the world.

The first nursing home for the dying was opened in Dublin, Ireland, by an order of nuns called the Irish Sisters of Charity, in the middle of the 19th century. In 1905 a similar home, St Joseph's Hospice, run by the same order, was opened in London.

The modern hospice movement was founded by Dame Cicely Saunders at St Christopher's Hospice, Sydenham, on the outskirts of London, some 30 years ago. Dame Cicely, who was a nurse and a social worker before she qualified in medicine, became the first full-time medical director of St Joseph's Hospice, where she began her research into methods of pain control and the special needs of dying patients.

She founded St Christopher's Hospice in 1967 as a place where effective care of those who are dying could be both practised and taught, and where research could be carried out that would develop this important field of medicine and nursing.

Hospices are generally calm and tranquil places where the symptoms of those who are dying can be brought under control, and their lives made easier. Patients often come in for short periods of medical and nursing care to enable them to go home and stay with their families. Hospice nurses visit them regularly to give them and their relatives care and support, and reassure them that they can go back into the hospice if they need to.

The atmosphere of a hospice is usually frank, open and compassionate. Patients are encouraged to discuss their problems with medical and nursing staff at any time, and often give each other support. The staff also care for bereaved relatives and help them through their grief.

From Britain, which now has a number of hospices funded jointly by charity and the state health system, the philosophy of hospice care has spread to more than 60 countries. Hospices and special units for what is called 'palliative care' (relief of symptoms) exist in almost every country in the Western world.

## Cancer nursing and natural therapy

Cancer nursing and 'palliative care' have become specialized branches of nursing. There is an International Society for Nurses in Cancer Care, with branches throughout the world (except for developing (Third World) countries where palliative care is seen as a luxury), and cancer nurses work in hospitals, nursing homes, and patients' homes, supporting them at all stages of their disease.

So many cancer nurses are aware of the value of natural therapies in palliative care these days that they have trained in them extensively and practise them alongside the more conventional methods of treatment – and often in preference to them. As many as 90 per cent of hospices in Britain, for example, are estimated to use natural therapies in palliative care, especially to help with pain and emotional distress.

Care of the dying is one of the most important and sensitive areas of medicine and nursing, and it is one in which the natural therapies have shown themselves to be particularly effective in relieving the suffering of cancer patients, and helping them to a peaceful end.

# CHAPTER 10

# How to find and choose a natural therapist

*Tips and guidelines for finding reliable help*

It is much easier now to find the right therapist than it was even a few years ago – but it is still not easy enough. The sheer variety of therapies is bewildering in itself and in many countries natural therapists are still not fully organized. There is no shortage of directories and advertisements but it is difficult from lists alone to know who to rely on for what. So how do you find a therapist you can trust?

### Starting the search: local sources

As we have seen, many of the natural therapies highlighted in this book have their roots in antiquity. Some have existed for as long as human beings have lived on earth, and finding a good practitioner has been a matter of tuning in to the community 'bush telegraph'. Word of mouth is still the best way to find the right practitioner.

Speak to anyone whose opinion you respect, especially if he or she is also a fellow sufferer. (You will also want to know who should be avoided, and which therapies might not help you at all.) If this does not work there are several other ways you can try.

## Doctors' clinics and medical centres

If you need help urgently you must see your family doctor. It has already been explained in this book that your condition can decline quickly without the proper treatment. If you ask about natural therapies at your first appointment, be prepared to hear anything from a dire warning to a recommendation that you might try a natural therapist once your condition is stable. Alternatively you could go to a 'holistic' specialist cancer help centre such as the one in Bristol, England (*see* appendix A).

## Natural health centres

Your nearest natural health centre should be happy to advise you. Your first impressions will often be a good guide to the quality of service they provide. Are the staff well informed and friendly? Is the place clean and comfortable? Does the atmosphere make you feel comfortable from the moment you walk in? It should. It matters. You are bringing them your trust and your custom and both should be treated with the utmost respect.

A good centre should have plenty of information explaining the therapies and introducing the practitioners. In a well-run practice the receptionist or owner will know all about the different therapies on offer. It's a bad sign if they don't.

You may still be unsure after your first impressions whether to book in or not. If so, ask to meet the person who might be treating you, just to test the waters. This should be possible, even in a busy practice.

Don't start off by telling your full life history, but some practices do offer you this opportunity during a free consultation – usually 15 minutes – just to see whether you have come to the right place or not.

## *Local practitioners*

Practitioners tend to know who's who in the area, even in therapies other than their own. So if you know, say, a reflexologist, but want a homoeopath, ask for a recommendation. The same applies if you know a practitioner socially and so don't want to consult him or her professionally. Practitioners are usually happy to recommend someone else in the same field.

## *Healthfood stores and alternative bookshops*

The staff in these kinds of shops often have a good local knowledge as well as an interest in the subject of natural therapies. The shop may well have a noticeboard with local practitioners' business cards on it. Remember, though, the most experienced and well-established practitioners don't need this kind of advertising, so you might miss them altogether if you don't actually check up by asking.

## *Other sources of local knowledge*

Don't forget that your local pharmacist often has contacts with both conventional and natural therapists.

The local library or information centre may be another good source of contact, especially for finding self-help or support groups.

Computers (using a modem) can provide this type of information via the Internet system, and other sources worth trying are health farms, beauty therapists and citizens' advice bureaux.

## Wider sources of information

If you have no luck on a local level, don't give up – there are several more leads you can follow up at a national level.

## 'Umbrella' organizations

The natural therapies are increasingly coming together under 'umbrella' organizations that represent a therapy or range of therapies nationally under one banner or heading. These national umbrella organizations have lists of registered and approved practitioners, and in the case of the more established therapies (such as chiropractic) have their own regulatory bodies already in place.

It is better to phone than to write or fax because this should give you a good idea of how well organized the group is. You may find that the group you are contacting has several different associations under its banner. A small charge may be made for each association's register but if you can afford it get the lot and then make up your own mind.

## Newspapers, magazines and local directories

Many therapists advertise. If you find local practitioners this way it's a good idea to talk to them and check them out first.

## Checking professional organizations

Some organizations are genuine groups that really keep a check on their members, while others seem to spring up like weeds, apparently interested only in collecting membership fees and giving themselves credibility. This section helps you do your own weeding.

## Why do professional organizations exist?

The purposes of governing bodies for natural therapies are:

● to keep up-to-date lists of their members so you can check whether someone is really on their list or not

- to protect you by making sure that their members are fully trained, licensed and insured against accident, negligence and malpractice
- to give you someone to complain to if you are unhappy with any aspect of treatment you have received, and you can't sort the matter out with your therapist
- to protect their members by giving good ethical and legal advice
- to represent their members when laws which might affect them are being made
- to work towards improvements in education for their members both before and after qualifying
- to work towards greater awareness of the benefit of each therapy in conventional medical circles
- to improve public awareness of the benefit of each therapy

### Questions to ask professional organizations

A good organization will publish clear and simple information on its status and purposes along with its membership list. As they don't all do this you may find it useful to contact them again on receiving your list to ask the following:

- When was the association founded? (You may be reassured to hear it has been around for 50 years. If the association is new, however, don't reject it out of hand. Ask why it was formed – it may be innovative.)
- How many members does it have? (Size reflects public demand, as few therapists could survive in a therapy if there was no call for it. The bigger organizations generally have a better track record and greater public acceptance, but a small association may just reflect the fact that the therapy is very specialized or still in its infancy – not necessarily a bad thing.)

- When was the therapy that it represents started?
- Is it a charity or educational trust – with a proper constitution, management committee, and published accounts – or is it a private limited company? (Charities have to be non-profitmaking, work in the public interest, and be open to inspection at any time. Private companies don't.)
- Is it part of a larger network of organizations? (If so, this implies it is interested in progress by consensus with other groups, and not just in furthering its own aims. By and large, groups that go their own way are more suspect than those that join in.)
- Does the organization have a code of ethics (upholding standards of professional behaviour) and disciplinary procedures? If so, what are they?
- How do its members gain admission to its register? Is it linked to only one school? (Beware of associations whose heads are also head of the school they represent: unbiased help may be in short supply with this type of 'one man band'.)
- Do members have to have proof of professional indemnity insurance? This should cover:
  - accidental damage to yourself or your property while you are on the practitioner's work premises
  - negligence (either the failure of the practitioner to exercise the 'duty of care' owed to you, or his or her falling below the standards of clinical competence demanded by his or her qualifications, bringing about an overall worsening of your problem)
  - malpractice (a 'falling from grace' over professional conduct, involving, for example, dishonesty, sexual misconduct or breach of confidence – your personal details should *never* be discussed with a third person without your permission)

## Checking training and qualifications

If you have reassured yourself so far but are still puzzled by what the training actually involves, ask a few more questions:

- How long is the training?
- Is it full or part time?
- If it is part time but shorter than a full-time course leading to the same qualifications, does the time spent at lectures and in clinic add up to the same as a full-time course overall? (In other words, is it a short cut?)
- Does it include seeing patients under supervision at a college clinic and in real practices?
- What do the initials after the therapist's name mean? Do they denote simply membership of an organization or do they indicate in-depth study?
- Are the qualifications recognized? If so, by whom? (This is becoming more relevant as the therapy organizations group together and start to form state-recognized registers in many countries. But the really important thing to know is if the qualifications are recognized by an independent outside assessment authority.)

## Making the choice

Making the final choice is a matter of using a combination of common sense and intuition, and finding the resolution to give someone a try. Don't forget that the most important part of the whole process is your resolve to feel better, to have more control over your state of health, and hopefully to see an improvement in your condition. The next most important part is that you feel comfortable with your chosen therapist.

**What is it like seeing a natural therapist?**

Since most natural therapists, even in those countries with state health systems, still work privately, there is no established common pattern.

Although they may all share more or less a belief in the principles outlined in chapter 6, you are liable to come across individuals from all walks of life. You will find as much variety in dress, thinking and behaviour as there are fashions, ranging from the formal and sophisticated to the absolutely informal.

Equally, you will find their premises very different. Some will present a 'brass plaque' image, working in a clinic with a receptionist and brisk efficiency, while others will see you in their living room surrounded by plants and domestic clutter.

Remember, though, that while image may be some indication of status, it is little guarantee of ability. You are as likely to find a therapist of quality working from home as in a formal clinic.

Some characteristics, however, and probably the most important ones, are common to all natural therapists:

● They will give you far more time than you are used to with a family doctor. An initial consultation will rarely last less than an hour, and is often longer. They will ask you all about yourself so they can form a proper understanding of what makes you tick and what may be the fundamental cause(s) of your problem.
● You will have to pay for any remedies they prescribe, and they may well sell you these from their own stocks. They will also charge you for their time – though many therapists offer reduced fees for deserving cases or for people who genuinely cannot afford the full fee.

## Sensible precautions

- Be sceptical of anyone who 'guarantees' you a cure. No one (not even doctors) can do that.
- Query any attempt to book you in for a course of treatment. Your response to any natural therapy is highly individual. Of course, if the practice is a busy one, booking ahead for one or two sessions might be sensible. You should be able to cancel without penalty any sessions which prove unnecessary (but remember to give at least 24 hours' notice: some practitioners will charge you if you don't give enough notice).
- No ethical therapist will ask for fees in advance of treatment unless for special tests or medicines – and even this is unusual. If you are asked for 'down payments' of any sort, ask exactly what they are for. If you don't like the reasons, don't pay.
- Be wary if you are not asked about your existing medication and try to give precise answers when you are asked. Be especially wary if the therapist tells you to stop or change any medically prescribed drug without talking to your doctor first. (A responsible doctor should also be happy to discuss you and your medication with a therapist.)
- Note the quality of the therapist's touch if you choose any of the relaxation or manipulation techniques such as massage, aromatherapy or osteopathy. It should never be lingering or suggestive. If, for any reason, the therapist wants to touch you on the breasts or genitals, your permission should be sought first.
- If the practitioner is of the opposite sex you are entitled to have someone of your choice in the room at the same time. Be immediately suspicious if this is not allowed. Ethical therapists will not refuse this sort of request, and if they do, it is probably best to have nothing more to do with them.

## What to do if things go wrong

A practitioner is in a position of trust, and is charged with a duty of care to you at all times. It does not mean you are 'entitled' to a 'cure' just because you've paid for treatment, but if you feel you are being treated unfairly, incompetently or unethically, you have several options:

- Tackle the matter at the source of the problem, with your practitioner, either verbally or in writing.
- If he or she works in a place such as a clinic, health farm or sports centre, tell the management. They also have a duty to protect the public and should treat complaints seriously and discreetly.
- Contact the practitioner's professional organization. It should have an independent panel that investigates complaints fully and disciplines its members.
- If the offence committed is a criminal one report it to the police (but be prepared for the problem of proving one person's word against another's).
- If you feel compensation is due see a lawyer for advice.

Short of a public court case, the worst thing for a truly incompetent or unethical practitioner is bad publicity. Tell everyone about your experiences. People only need to hear the same sort of comments from a few different sources and the practitioner will probably sink without trace. Before you do so, though, try the other measures first and give yourself time to consider things calmly. Vengeance is not very healing.

*A word of warning* Don't make malicious allegations without good reason. Such actions are themselves a criminal offence in most countries and you could end up in more trouble than the practitioner.

## Summary

The reality is that there are few real crooks or charlatans in natural therapy. Despite the myth, there is little real money in it unless the therapist is very busy – and the chances are high that a busy therapist is a good one. Remember that no one can know everything and no specialist qualified in any field has to get 100 per cent in the exams to be able to practise. Perfection is an ideal, not a reality, and to err is human.

It is very much for this reason that taking control of your own health is perhaps the single most important lesson underlying this book. Taking control means taking responsibility for the choices you make, and this is one of the most significant factors in successful treatment.

No one but you can decide on a practitioner and no one but you can determine if that practitioner is any good or not. You will know this very easily, and probably very quickly, by the way you feel about the person and the therapy, and by whether or not you get any better.

If you are not happy, the decision is yours whether to stay or move on – and continue moving until you find the right therapist for you. Don't despair if you don't find the right person first time. There is almost bound to be the right person for you somewhere and your determination to get well is the best resource you have for finding that person.

Above all, bear in mind that many people who have taken this route before you have not only been helped beyond their most optimistic dreams, but have also found a close and trusted helper who will assist in times of trouble – and who may even become a friend for life.

# Useful organizations

*The following listing of organizations is for information only and does not imply any endorsement, nor do the organizations listed necessarily agree with the views expressed in this book.*

## INTERNATIONAL

**International Federation of Practitioners of Natural Therapeutics**
10 Copse Close
Sheet
Petersfield
Hampshire GU31 4DL, UK.
Tel 01730 266790
Fax 01730 260058

## AUSTRALASIA

**Acupuncture Ethics and Standards Organization**
PO Box 84
Merrylands
New South Wales 2160,
Australia.

**Australian Association for Hospice and Palliative Care**
PO Box 1200
North Fitzroy
Victoria 3068, Australia.
Tel 3 486 2666
Fax 3 482 5094

**Australian Cancer Society Inc.**
153 Dowling Street
Woolloomooloo
New South Wales 2011
Australia.
Tel 2 358 2066
Fax 2 356 4558

**Australian Federation of Aromatherapists**
35 Bydown Street
Neutral Bay
New South Wales 2089
Australia.

**Australian Natural Therapists Association**
PO Box 308
Melrose Park
South Australia 5039, Australia.
Tel 8 297 9533
Fax 8 297 0003

**Australian Traditional Medicine Society**
PO Box 442
Suite 3, First Floor
120 Blaxland Road
Ryde
New South Wales 2112
Australia.
Tel 2 808 2825
Fax 2 809 7570

**Cancer Society of New Zealand Inc**
PO Box 12145
Wellington, New Zealand.
Tel 4 473 6409
Fax 4 499 0849

**New Zealand Natural Health Practitioners Accreditation Board**
PO Box 37-491
Auckland
New Zealand
Tel 9 625 9966

**New Zealand Register of Acupuncturists**
PO Box 9950
Wellington 1
New Zealand.

**The Gawler Foundation**
Yarra Valley Living Centre
PO Box 77G
Yarra Junction
Victoria 3979, Australia.
Tel 5 967 1730

## NORTH AMERICA

**American Academy of Medical Preventics**
6151 West Century Boulevard
Suite 1114
Los Angeles
California 90045, USA.
Tel 213 645 5350

**American Aromatherapy Association**
PO Box 3609
Culver City
California 90231, USA.

**American Association of Acupuncture and Oriental Medicine**
National Acupuncture Headquarters
1424 16th Street NW, Suite 501
Washington DC 200 36, USA.

**American Cancer Society**
1599 Clifton Road NE
Atlanta
Georgia 30329, USA.
Tel 404 320 3333
Fax 404 325 0230

**American Holistic Medical Association**
6728 Old McLean Village Drive
McLean, VA 22101, USA
Tel 703 556 9222

**Canadian Cancer Society**
10 Alcorn Avenue, Suite 200
Toronto
Ontario M4V 3B1, Canada.
Tel 416 961 7223
Fax 416 961 4189

**Canadian Holistic Medical Association**
700 Bay Street
PO Box 101, Suite 604
Toronto
Ontario M5G 1Z6, Canada.
Tel 416 599 0447

**National Cancer Institute**
Building 31, Room 10A24
9000 Rockville Pike
Bethesda
Maryland 20892, USA.
Tel 301 496 5583
Fax 301 402 2594

**National Coalition for Cancer Survivalship**
1010 Wayne Avenue
Silver Spring
Maryland 20910, USA.
Tel 301 650 8868.

**SOUTHERN AFRICA**

**Cancer Association of South Africa**
PO Box 2000
Johannesburg
South Africa.
Tel 11 616 7662

**South Africa Homoeopaths, Chiropractors and Allied Professions Board**
PO Box 17055
0027 Groenkloof
South Africa.
Tel 12 466 455

**UK & EIRE**

**British Association for Counselling**
1 Regent Place
Rugby
Warwickshire CV21 2PJ
England.
Tel 01788 578328

**British Association for Cancer United Patients (BACUP)**
3 Bath Place
Rivington Street
London EC2A 3JR, England.
Tel (Cancer Information Service freeline) 0800 181199, (Cancer Counselling Service) 0171 696 9000

**Breast Cancer Care**
210 New Kings Road
London SW6 4NZ, England.
Tel helplines (nationwide freeline) 0500 245 345, (London) 0171 867 1103

**Bristol Cancer Help Centre**
Grove House
Cornwallis Grove
Clifton
Bristol BS8 4PG, England.
Tel 0117 9743216

**British Colostomy Association**
15 Station Road
Reading
Berkshire RG1 1LG, England.
Tel 01734 391537

**British Complementary Medicine Association**
39 Prestbury Road
Cheltenham
Gloucestershire GL25 2PT
England.
Tel 01242 226770

**British Holistic Medical Association**
Royal Shrewsbury Hospital South
Shrewsbury
Shropshire SY3 8XF, England.
Tel 01743 261155
Fax 01743 353637

**Cancer Care Society**
21 Zetland Road
Redland
Bristol BS6 7AH, England.
Tel 0117 9427419

**CancerLink**
17 Britannia Street
London WC1X 9JN, England.
Tel (Cancer Information Service)
0171 833 2451

**Cancer Relief Macmillan Fund**
Anchor House
15-19 Britten Street
London SW3 3TZ, England.
Tel 0171 351 7811

**Cancer Research Campaign**
10 Cambridge Terrace
London NW1 4JL, England.
Tel 0171 224 1333
Fax 0171 487 4310

**Carers' National Association**
20-25 Glasshouse Yard
London EC1A 4JS, England.
Tel 0171 490 8818

**Confederation of Healing Organisations**
Suite J, The Red & White House
113 High Street
Berkhamsted
Hertfordshire HP4 2DJ, England.
Tel 01442 870660

**Council for Complementary and Alternative Medicine**
179 Gloucester Place
London NW1 6DX, England.
Tel 0171 724 9103
Fax 0171 724 5330

**Counselling Information Scotland**
Health Education Board for
Scotland
Woodburn House
Canaan Lane
Edinburgh EH10 4SG, Scotland.
Tel 0131 452 8989

**European Therapy Studies Institute**
Henry House
189 Heene Road
Worthing
West Sussex BN11 4NN
England.
Tel/fax 01903 236179.

**Hodgkin's Disease and Lymphoma Association**
PO Box 275
Haddenham
Aylesbury
Buckinghamshire HP17 8JJ
England.
Tel 01844 291500

**Hospice Information Service**
St Christopher's Hospice
51-59 Lawrie Park Road
Sydenham
London SE26 6DZ, England.

**Imperial Cancer Research Fund**
PO Box 123
Lincoln's Inn Fields
London WC2A 3PX, England.
Tel 0171 242 0200
Fax 0171 269 3262

**Institute for Complementary Medicine**
PO Box 194
London SE16 1QZ, England.
Tel 0171 237 5165
Fax 0171 237 5175

**Irish Cancer Society**
5 Northumberland Road
Dublin 4, Eire.
Tel 1 668 1855, (National helpline) 1 800 200 700

**Leukaemia Care Society**
14 Kingfisher Court
Venny Bridge
Pinhoe
Exeter
Devon EX4 8JN, England.
Tel 01392 464848

**Marie Curie Cancer Care**
28 Belgrave Square
London SW1X 8QG, England.
Tel 0171 235 3325

**National Association of Laryngectomee Clubs**
Ground Floor
6 Rickett Street
London SW6 1RU, England.
Tel 0171 381 9993

**Tak Tent Cancer Support**
The Western Infirmary Block
20 Western Court
100 University Place
Glasgow G12 6SQ, Scotland.
Tel 0141 211 1930

**Tenovus Cancer Information Centre**
142 Whitchurch Road
Cardiff CF4 3NA, Wales.
Tel 01222 619846, (National freephone helpline) 0800 526 527

**Ulster Cancer Foundation**
40-42 Eglantine Avenue
Belfast BT96 6DX
Northern Ireland.
Tel 01232 663281, (National helpline) 01232 663439

**Women's Health Information Centre**
52-54 Featherstone Street
London EC1Y 8RT, England.
Tel 0171 251 6580

**Women's Nationwide Cancer Control Campaign**
Suna House
128-130 Curtain Road
London EC2A 3AR, England.
Tel 0171 729 4688, (Helpline) 0171 729 2229

**Yoga Biomedical Trust**
PO Box 140
Cambridge, England.
CB1 1 PU

# Useful further reading

*Antioxidant Nutrition*, Rita Greer and Robert Woodward (Souvenir Press, UK, 1995)

*Choices in Healing*, Michael Lerner (MIT, USA/UK, 1994)

*Encyclopaedia of Natural Medicine*, Michael Murray and Joseph Pizzorno (Macdonald Optima, UK, 1990)

*Healing and the Mind*, Bill Moyers (Doubleday, USA, 1993)

*Let's Get the Fear Out of Cancer*, Vernon Templemore (Gateway Books, UK, 1991)

*Living with Cancer*, Jenny Bryan and Joanna Lyall (Penguin, UK, 1987)

*Love, Medicine and Miracles*, Bernie Siegel (Harper & Row, USA, 1986/Arrow, UK, 1988)

*Massage for People with Cancer*, Patricia McNamara (Wandsworth Cancer Support Centre, UK, 1994)

*Mind-Body Medicine: How to Use Your Mind for Better Health*, eds Daniel Goleman and Joel Gurin (Consumer Reports Books, USA, 1993)

*Miracles Do Happen*, C Norman Shealy (Element Books, UK/USA, 1995)

*Nutritional Medicine*, Stephen Davies and Alan Stewart (Pan Books, UK, 1987)

*Nutrition and Cancer*, Sandra Goodman (Green Library, UK, 1995)

*Reader's Digest Family Guide to Alternative Medicine*, ed Patrick Pietroni (The Reader's Digest Association, UK/USA/South Africa/Australia, 1991)

*Remarkable Recovery*, Caryle Hirshberg and Marc Ian Barasch (Riverhead Books, USA/Headline, UK, 1995)

*The Bristol Experience*, Liz Hodgkinson and Jane Metcalfe (Vermilion Books, UK, 1995)

*The Healing Foods Book*, Rosy Daniel (Thorsons, UK, 1996)

*Wells' Supportive Therapies in Health Care*, ed Richard Wells with Vera Tschudin (Baillière Tindall, UK, 1994)

*You Don't Have to Feel Unwell*, Robin Needes (Gateway Books, UK, 1994)

# Index